Obstetric Anatomy

Normal and Abnormal Labor

Akmal El-Mazny

CONTENTS

<u>INTRODUCTION</u>

As the mechanism of labor is essentially a process of accommodation between the fetus and the passage through which it must pass, it is apparent that obstetrics lacked a scientific foundation until the anatomy of the bony pelvis and of the ' soft parts connected with it was clearly understood (J. Whitridge Williams).

The WHO defines normal birth as: spontaneous in onset, low-risk throughout labor and delivery, the infant is born spontaneously in the vertex position between 37 and 42 weeks of pregnancy, and after birth, mother and infant are in good condition.

The three main factors associated with abnormal labor are the power (inadequate uterine contractions), the passage (abnormal pelvic anatomy), and the passenger (eg, macrosomia or malpresentation).

This book provides a comprehensive review of maternal and fetal obstetric anatomy, emphasizing the mechanism and management of normal and abnormal labor, which will be of immense value for obstetricians and allied health professionals.

OBSTETRIC ANATOMY

ANATOMY OF FEMALE PELVIS

The female bony pelvis is divided into:

False pelvis (above the pelvic brim): Has no obstetric importance.

- True pelvis (below the pelvic brim): Related to the child-birth.

Composed of inlet, cavity, and outlet.

Pelvic Inlet (Brim)

Boundaries

- Sacral promontory.

- Alae of the sacrum.

- Sacroiliac joints.

- Iliopectineal lines.

- Iliopectineal eminencies.

- Upper border of the superior pubic rami.

- Pubic tubercles.

- Pubic crests.

- Upper border of symphysis pubis.

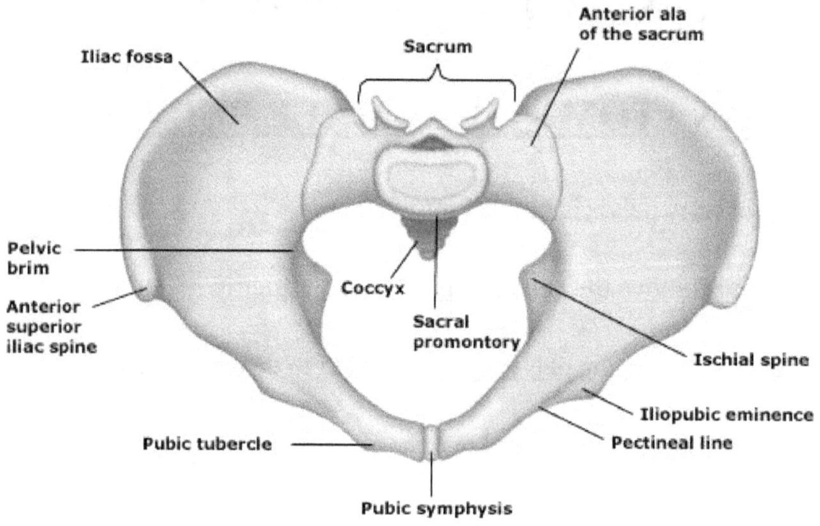

Pelvic Inlet

<u>Diameters</u>

<u>Antero-Posterior Diameters</u>

<u>Anatomical Antero-Posterior Diameter = True Conjugate (11 cm)</u>

From the tip of the sacral promontory to the upper border of the symphysis pubis.

<u>Obstetric Conjugate (10.5 cm)</u>

From the tip of the sacral promontory to the most bulging point on the back of symphysis pubis which is about 1 cm below its upper border.

It is the shortest antero-posterior diameter.

<u>Diagonal Conjugate (12.5 cm)</u>

From the tip of sacral promontory to lower border of symphysis pubis.

Can be measured by vaginal examination.

<u>External Conjugate (20 cm)</u>

From the depression below last lumbar spine to the upper anterior margin of symphysis pubis measured from outside by the pelvimeter.

It has not a true obstetric importance.

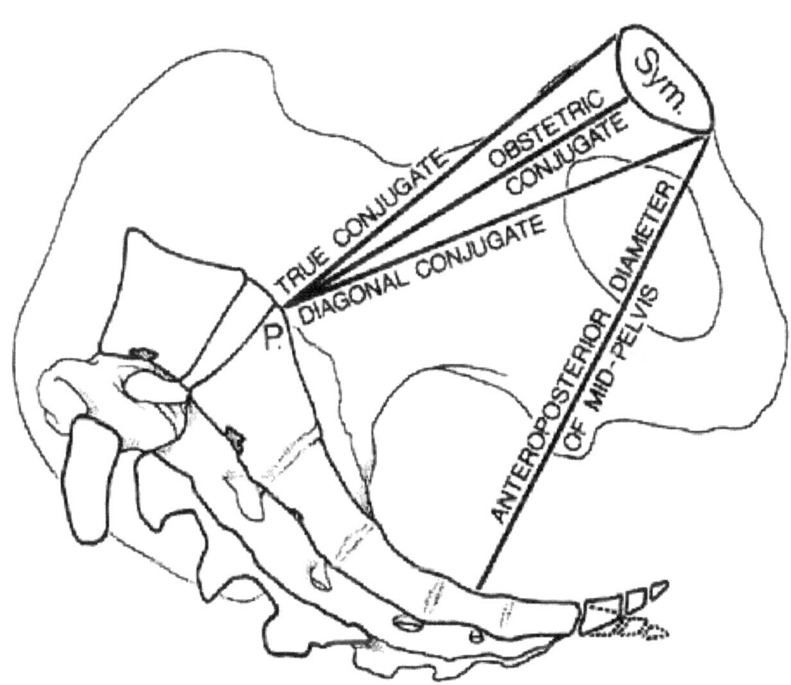

Antero-Posterior Diameters

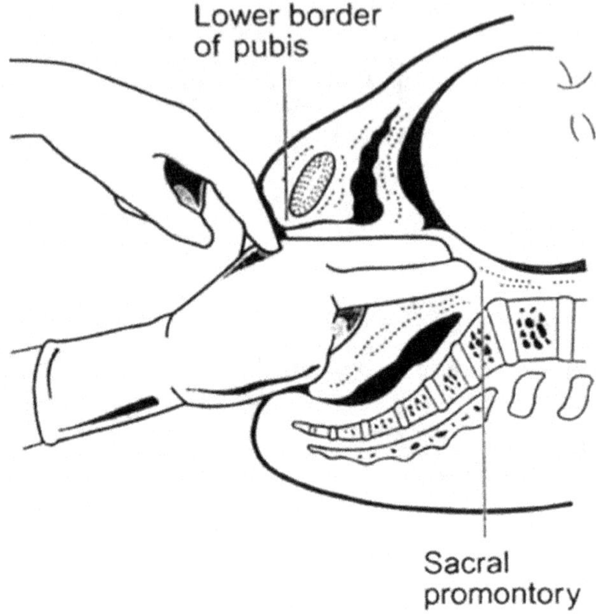

Diagonal Conjugate

<u>Transverse Diameters</u>

<u>Anatomical Transverse Diameter (13 cm)</u>

Between the farthest two points on the iliopectineal lines.

It lies 4 cm anterior to the promontory and 7 cm behind the symphysis.

It is the largest diameter in the pelvis.

<u>Obstetric Transverse Diameter (11-12 cm)</u>

It bisects the true conjugate and is slightly shorter than the anatomical transverse diameter.

Oblique Diameters

<u>Right Oblique Diameter (12 cm)</u>

From the right sacroiliac joint to the left iliopectineal eminence.

<u>Left Oblique Diameter (12 cm)</u>

From the left sacroiliac joint to the right iliopectineal eminence.

<u>Sacro-Cotyloid Diameters (9-9.5 cm)</u>

From promontory of the sacrum to right and left iliopectineal eminence.

Pelvic Cavity

The roof is the plane of pelvic brim.

The floor is the plane of least pelvic dimension.

Pelvic Outlet

Anatomical Outlet

It is lozenge-shaped bounded by:

– Lower border of symphysis pubis.

– Pubic arch.

– Ischial tuberosities.

– Sacrotuberous and sacrospinous ligaments.

– Tip of the coccyx.

Obstetric Outlet

It is a segment, the boundaries of which are:

– The roof: the plane of least pelvic dimension.

– The floor: the anatomical outlet.

– Anteriorly: the lower border of symphysis pubis.

– Posteriorly: the coccyx.

– Laterally: the ischial spines.

Diameters of Pelvic Outlet

Antero-Posterior Diameters

Anatomical Antero-Posterior Diameter (11cm)

From the tip of the coccyx to the lower border of symphysis pubis.

Obstetric Antero-Posterior Diameter (13 cm)

From the tip of the sacrum to the lower border of symphysis pubis as the coccyx moves backwards during the second stage of labor.

Transverse Diameters

Bituberous Diameter (11 cm)

Between the inner aspects of the ischial tuberosities.

Bispinous Diameter (10.5 cm)

Between the tips of ischial spines.

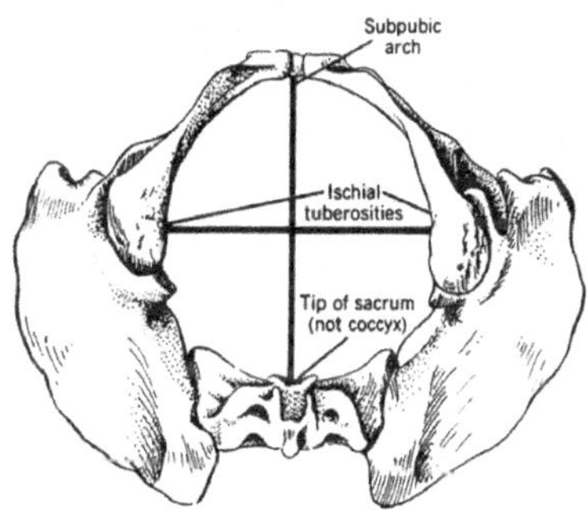
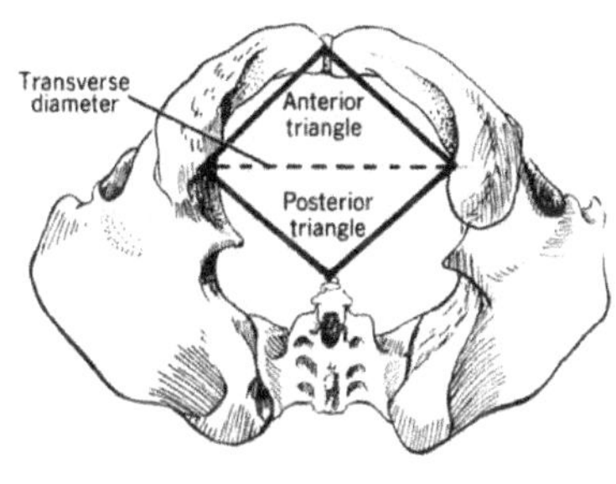

Pelvic Outlet

Pelvic Planes

These are imaginary planes lie as follow:

Plane of Pelvic Inlet

Passing with the boundaries of pelvic brim and making an angle of 55° with the horizon (angle of pelvic inclination).

Plane of Mid-Cavity = Plane of Greatest Pelvic Dimensions

Passes between the middle of the posterior surface of the symphysis pubis and the junction between 2nd and 3rd sacral vertebrae.

It is a round plane with diameter of 12.5 cm.

It is the widest part of the pelvic cavity.

Internal rotation of the head occurs when the biparietal diameter occupies this wide pelvic plane.

Plane of Obstetric Outlet = Plane of Least Pelvic Dimensions

Passes from the lower border of the symphysis pubis anteriorly, to the ischial spines laterally, to the tip of the sacrum posteriorly.

Plane of Anatomical Outlet

Passes with the boundaries of anatomical outlet.

Consists of 2 triangular planes with one base (the bituberous diameter):

– Anterior sagittal plane: Its apex at the lower border of symphysis pubis.

– Posterior sagittal plane: Its apex at the tip of the coccyx.

Anterior Sagittal Diameter (6-7 cm)

From the lower border of the symphysis pubis to the centre of the bituberous diameter.

Posterior Sagittal Diameter (7.5-10 cm)

From the tip of the sacrum to the centre of the bituberous diameter.

Types of Female Pelvis

– Gynecoid pelvis (50%): It is the normal female type.

– Anthropoid pelvis (25%): It is ape-like type.

– Android pelvis (20%): It is a male type.

– Platypelloid pelvis (5%): It is a flat female type.

– Mixed type (intermediates).

	Gynecoid	Anthropoid	Android	Platypelloid
Pelvic inlet Transverse diameter		Narrow		
AP diameter		Wide		Narrow
Forepelvis	Wide	Divergent	Narrow	Straight
Pelvic midcavity Side walls	Straight	Narrow	Convergent	Wide
Inclination of sacrum		Wide	Forward	Narrow
Pelvic outlet Subpubic arch	Wide		Narrow	Wide

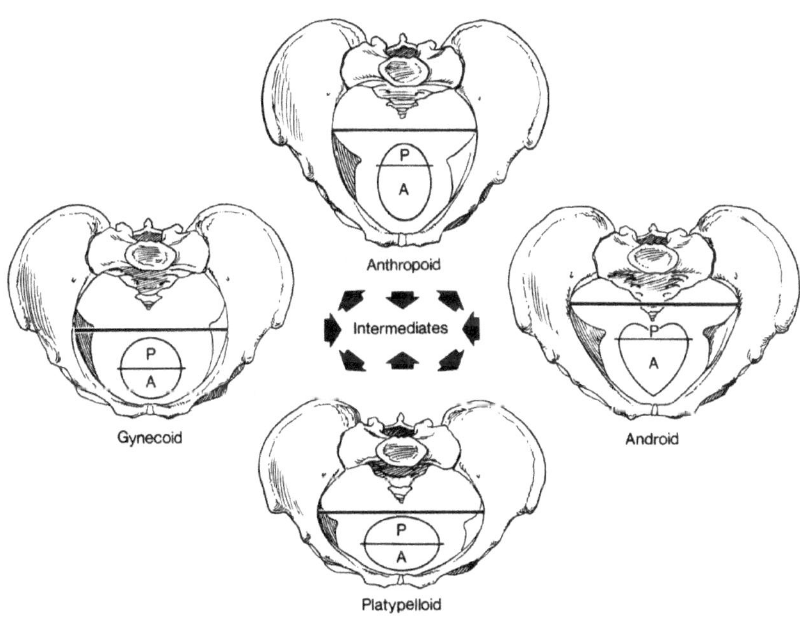

Types of Female Pelvis

ANATOMY OF FETAL SKULL

Fetal skull consists of 3 parts separated by sutures and fontanelles:

−Base: from the chin to the foramen magnum.

−Face: from the chin to the root of the nose and supraorbital margins.

−Vault: consists of three regions:

<u>Brow</u>

From the root of the nose and supraorbital margins to the anterior fontanelle (bregma) and coronal sutures.

It includes the 2 frontal bones separated by the frontal suture.

<u>Vertex</u>

From the bregma and coronal sutures to the posterior fontanelle and lambdoid suture.

It consists of 2 parietal bones separated by the sagittal suture.

It is bounded laterally by the parietal eminences.

<u>Occiput</u>

From the posterior fontanelle and lambdoid suture to the foramen magnum.

<u>Sutures</u>

Frontal, sagittal, coronal, lambdoid and temporal sutures.

Fontanelles

Four fontanelles lie at the anterior and posterior end of the temporal sutures on each side, and have no obstetric importance.

The anterior and posterior fontanelles are important to diagnose:

– Vertex presentation.

– Position of the occiput.

– Degree of flexion of the head.

Anterior Fontanelle (Bregma)

– Large, and lozenge-shaped.

– Its floor is membranous.

– Surrounded by 4 bons (2 frontal and 2 parietal).

– The floor is completely ossified 1.5 years after birth.

  The surrounding bones are not overlapping during moulding.

Posterior Fontanelle (Lambda)

– Small and triangular.

– Its floor is bony.

– Surrounded by 3 bones (2 parietal and occipital).

– The floor is completely ossified at full term.

– The surrounding bones are overlapping during moulding.

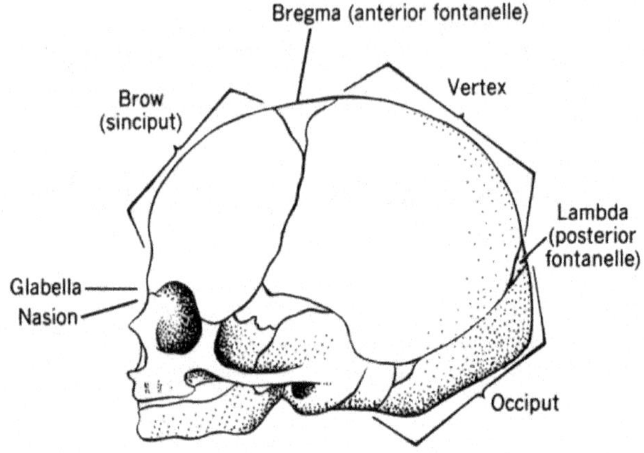

Anatomy of Fetal Skull

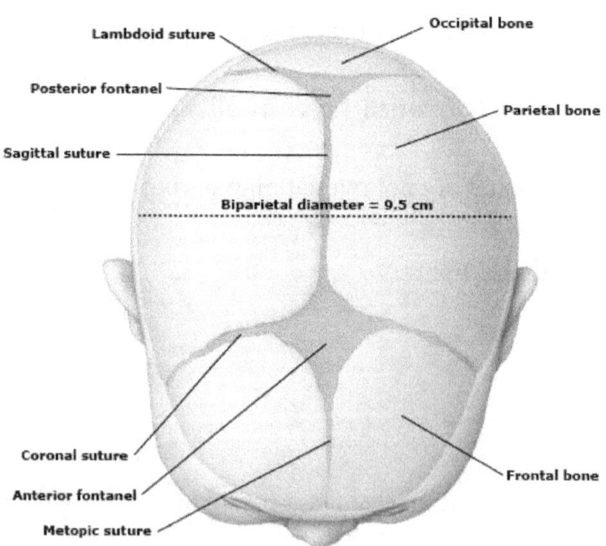

Sutures and Fontanelles

Diameters of Fetal Skull

Longitudinal Diameters

Suboccipito-Bregmatic (9.5 cm)

From below the occipital protuberance to the centre of bregma.

It is the engagement diameter in occipito-anterior with complete flexion.

Suboccipito-Frontal (10 cm)

From below the occipital protuberance to the anterior end of the bregma.

It is the diameter that distends the vulva in occipito anterior.

Occipito-Frontal (11.5 cm)

Form the occipital protuberance to the root of the nose.

It is the engagement diameter in occipito-posterior position.

It is the diameter that distends the vulva in face to pubis delivery.

Submento-Bregmatic (9.5 cm)

From the junction of the chin and neck to the centre of the bregma.

It is the engagement diameter in face presentation.

Submento-Vertical (11.5 cm)

From the junction of the chin and neck to the vertical point which is a point midway between anterior and posterior fontanelles.

It is the diameter that distends the vulva during face delivery.

Mento-Vertical (13.5 cm)

From the tip of the chin to the vertical point.

It is the engagement diameter when the head is partially extended (Brow presentation).

As it is longer than the largest diameter of the pelvic brim, the head cannot enter the pelvis.

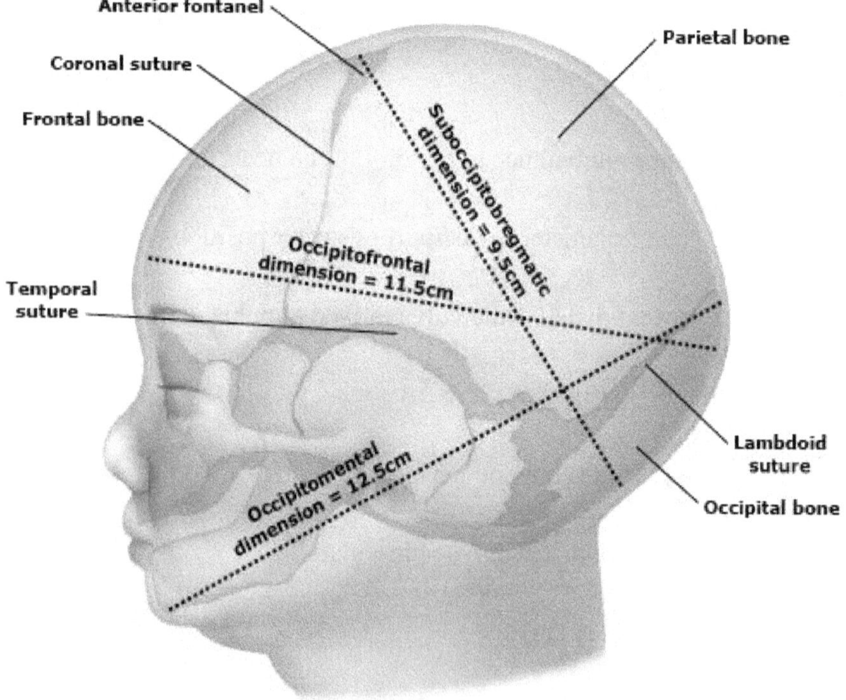

Longitudinal Diameters

Transverse Diameters

Biparietal Diameter (9.5 cm)

Between the 2 parietal eminencies.

Subparietal Supraparietal Diameter (9 cm)

From below one parietal eminence to above the opposite eminence.

Bitemporal Diameter (8 cm)

Between the anterior ends of the temporal sutures.

Bimastoid Diameter (7.5 cm)

Between the tips of the 2 mastoid processes.

Obstetric Terms

Presentation

The part of the fetus related to the pelvic brim and first felt during vaginal examination.

−Cephalic (96%):

  Vertex: when the head is flexed.

  Face: when the head is extended.

  Brow: when it is midway between flexion and extension.

– Breech (3.5%).

– Shoulder (0.5%).

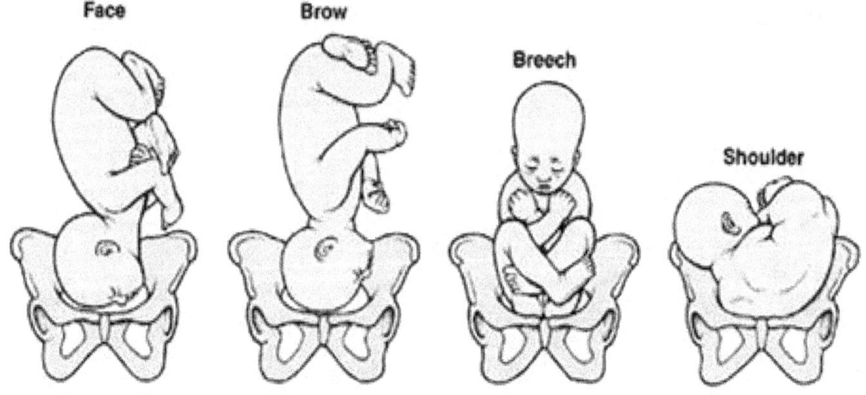

Abnormal Presentations

Cephalic presentation is the commonest as this makes the fetus more adapted to the pyriform-shaped uterus with the larger buttock in the wider fundus and the smaller head in the narrower lower part of the uterus.

Position

The relation of the fetal back to the right or left side of the mother and whether it is directed anteriorly or posteriorly.

The denominator: is a bony landmark on the presenting part used to denote the position.

– In vertex it is the occiput.

– In face it is the mentum (chin).

– In breech it is the sacrum.

– In shoulder it is the scapula.

In each presentation, except the shoulder, there are 8 positions.

In vertex presentation they are:

– Left occipito-anterior (LOA) = 60%.

– Right occipito-anterior (ROA) = 20%.

– Right occipito-posterior (ROP) = 15%.

– Left occipito-posterior (LOP).

– Left occipito-transverse (LOT).

– Right occipito-transverse (ROT).

– Direct occipito-anterior (DOA).

– Direct occipito-posterior (DOP).

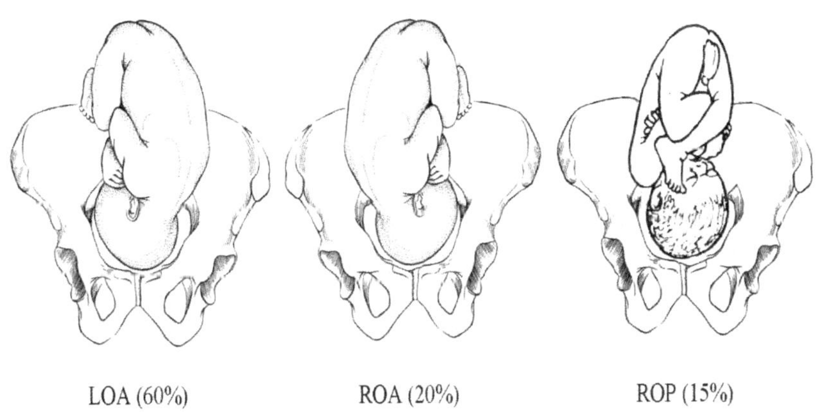

LOA (60%)   ROA (20%)   ROP (15%)

Vertex Presentation

OA positions are more common than OP positions because in OA positions the concavity of the anterior aspect of the fetus due to its flexion fits with the convexity of the vertebral column of the mother due to its lumbar lordosis.

LOA is more common than ROA, and ROP is more common than LOP as in LOA and ROP the head enters the pelvis in the right oblique diameter which is more favourable than the left oblique because:

– Anatomically, the right oblique is slightly longer than the left.

– The pelvic colon reduces the length of the left oblique.

Station

– Station 0 the vertex at the level of ischial spines (engagement).

– Station -1, -2 and -3 represent 1, 2 and 3 cm respectively above the level of ischial spines.

– Station +1, +2 and +3 represent 1, 2 and 3 cm respectively below the level of ischial spines.

Engagement

It is the passage of the widest transverse diameter of the presenting part, which is the biparietal in vertex presentation, through the pelvic inlet.

The engaged head cannot be easily grasped by the first pelvic grip, but it can be palpated by the second pelvic grip; 2/5 or less of the fetal head is felt above the symphysis pubis.

Vaginally, the vertex is felt at or below the level of ischial spines.

<u>In Primigravida</u>

Engagement of the head occurs in the last 3-4 weeks of pregnancy due to the tonicity of the abdominal and uterine muscles.

<u>In Multipara</u>

The head is usually engaged at the onset of labor or even at the beginning of the second stage due to less tonicity.

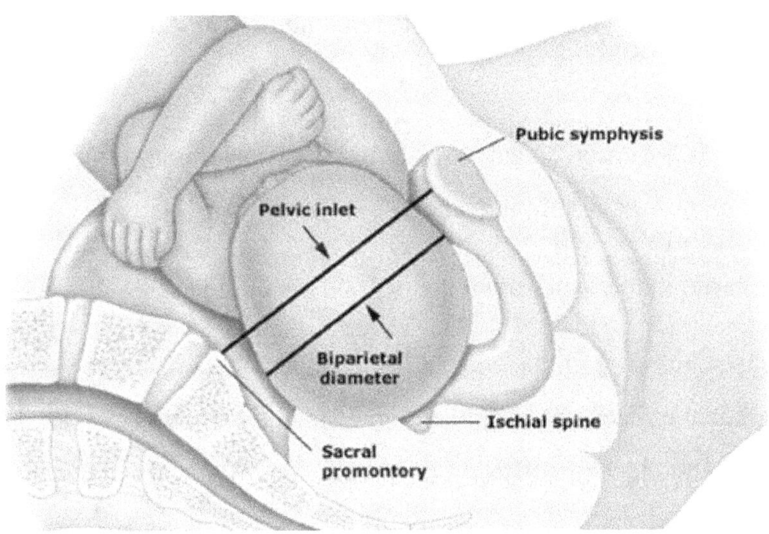

Engagement of Fetal Head

NORMAL LABOR

Labor is the physiological process by which a fetus is expelled from the uterus to the outside world.

Delivery means actual birth of the fetus.

The World Health Organization (WHO) defines normal birth as:

– Spontaneous in onset.

– Low-risk at the start of labor and remaining so throughout labor and delivery.

– The infant is born spontaneously in the vertex position between 37 and 42 completed weeks of pregnancy.

– After birth, mother and infant are in good condition.

Labor is achieved with changes in the biochemical connective tissue and with gradual effacement and dilatation of the uterine cervix as a result of uterine contractions of sufficient frequency, intensity, and duration.

The three main factors which affect the mechanics of active labor are the power, the passage, and the passenger.

The onset of labor is defined as regular, painful uterine contractions resulting in progressive cervical effacement and dilatation.

Labor is divided into three main stages that delineate milestones in a continuous process: the first stage (cervical dilation), the second stage (delivery of the fetus), and the third stage (delivery of the placenta).

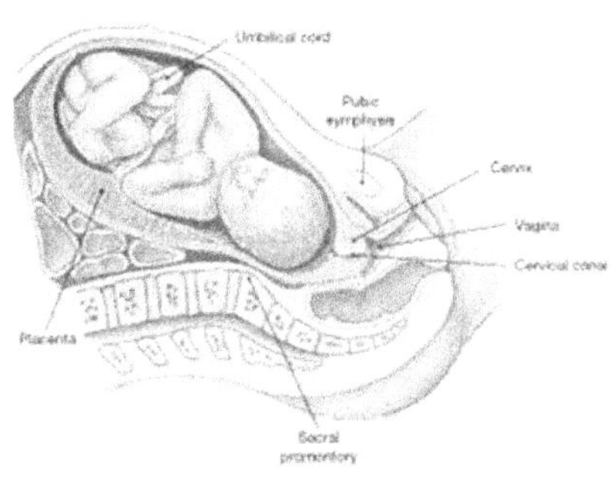

Pre-Labor

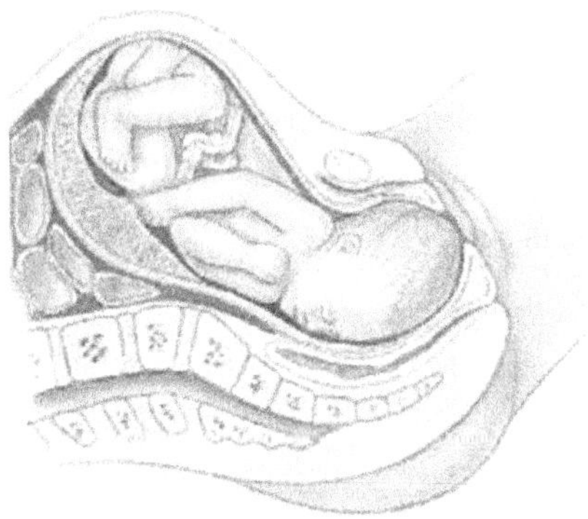

First Stage

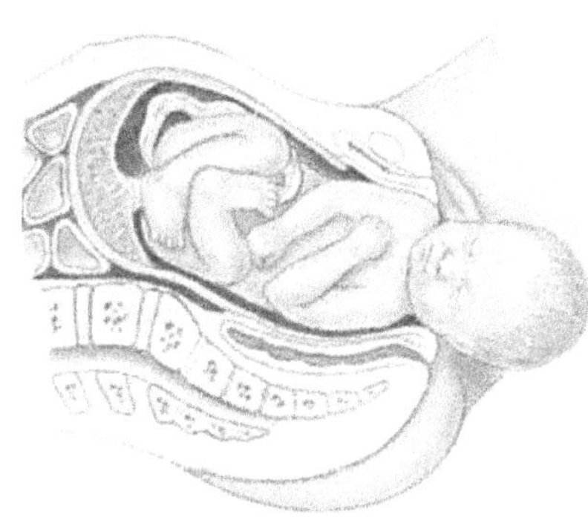

Second Stage

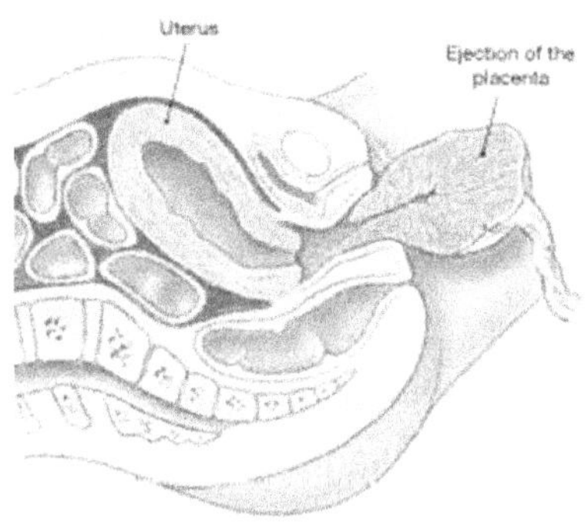

Third Stage

Stages of Labor

<u>FIRST STAGE OF LABOR</u>

It is the stage of cervical dilatation.

Starts with the onset of true labor pain.

Ends with full dilatation of the cervix i.e. 10 cm in diameter.

It takes about 10-14 hours in primigravida and about 6-8 hours in multipara.

<u>MECHANISM</u>

<u>Causes of Onset of Labor</u>

It is unknown but the following theories were postulated:

<u>Prostaglandins Theory</u>

Prostaglandins E2 and F2α are powerful stimulators of uterine muscle activity.

PGF2α was found to be increased in maternal and fetal blood as well as the amniotic fluid late in pregnancy and during labor.

<u>Oxytocin Theory</u>

Although oxytocin is a powerful stimulator of uterine contraction, its natural role in onset of labor is doubtful.

The secretion of oxytocinase enzyme from the placenta is decreased near term due to placental ischaemia leading to predominance of oxytocin action.

Estrogen Theory

During pregnancy, most of the estrogens are present in a binding form.

During the last trimester, more free estrogen appears increasing the excitability of the myometrium and prostaglandins synthesis.

Progesterone Withdrawal Theory

Before labor, there is a drop in progesterone synthesis leading to predominance of the excitatory action of estrogens.

Fetal Cortisol Theory

Increased cortisol production from the fetal adrenal gland before labor may influence its onset by increasing estrogen production from the placenta.

Anencephaly is associated with post-term pregnancy due to cortisol deficiency caused by lack of ACTH due to aplasia of the pituitary gland.

Uterine Distension Theory

Like any hollow organ in the body, when the uterus in distended to a certain limit, it starts to contract to evacuate its contents.

This explains the preterm labor in case of multiple pregnancy and polyhydramnios.

Stretch of the Lower Uterine Segment

Stretch of the lower uterine segment by the presenting part near term leads to reflex contraction of uterine muscle.

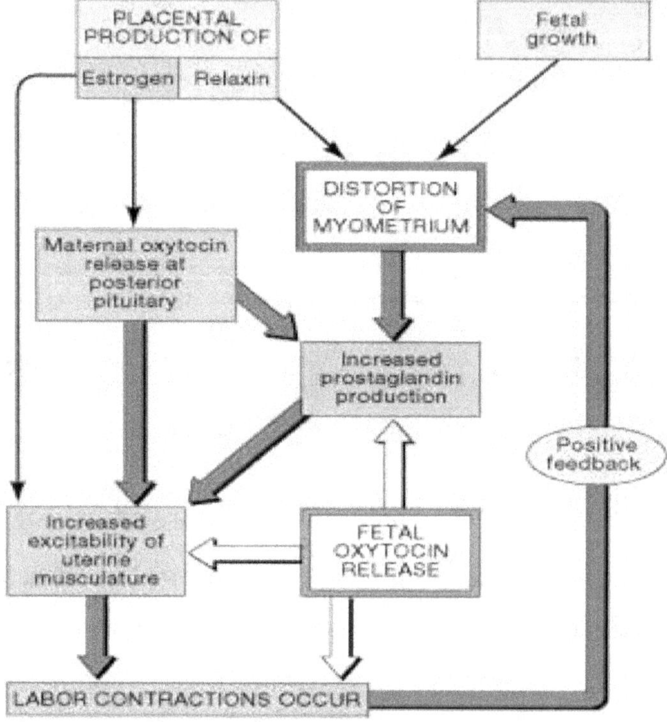

Causes of Onset of Labor

Causes of Cervical Dilatation

– Contraction and retraction of uterine musculature.

– Softness of the cervix which has occurred during pregnancy facilitates dilatation and effacement of the cervix.

– Mechanical pressure by the forebag of waters, if membranes still intact, or the presenting part, if they had ruptured; this in turn will release more prostaglandins which stimulate uterine contractions and cervical dilatation and effacement.

Mechanism of Cervical Dilatation

In Primigravida

The cervical canal dilates from above downwards i.e. from the internal os downwards to the external os, so its length shorts gradually to a thin rim of few millimetres continuous with the lower uterine segment.

This process is called effacement and expressed in percentage so when we say effacement is 50% it means that 50% of the cervical canal has been taken up.

Dilatation of the cervix (external os) starts after complete effacement of the cervix.

In Multipara

Effacement and dilatation occur simultaneously.

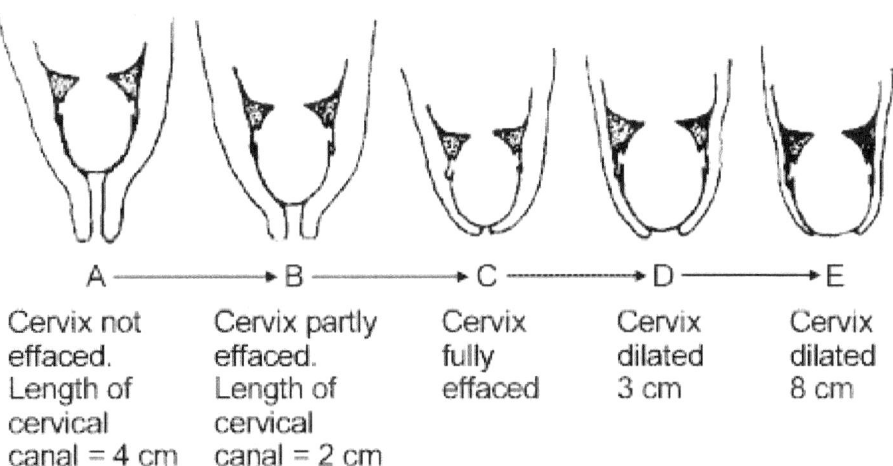

Effacement and Dilatation of the Cervix

Phases of Cervical Dilatation

Latent Phase

This is the first 3 cm of cervical dilatation which is slow takes about 8 hours in nulliparae and 4 hours in multiparae.

Active phase

– Acceleration phase.

– Maximum slope phase.

– Deceleration phase.

The normal rate of cervical dilatation in active phase is 1.2 cm / hour in primigravida and 1.5 cm / hour in multipara.

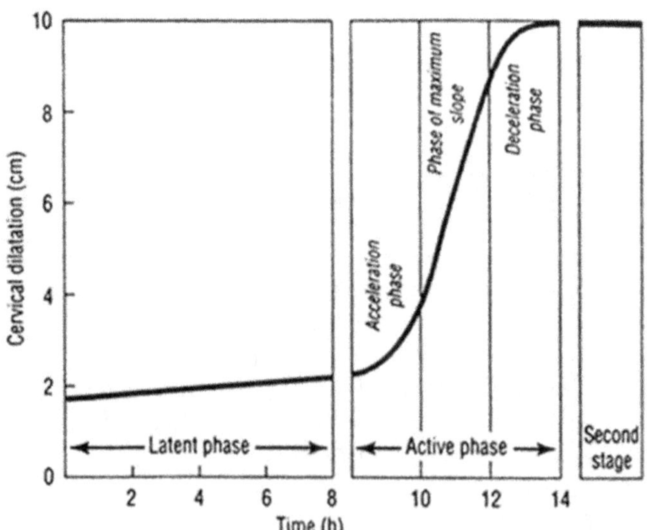

Friedman Labor Curve

MANAGEMENT

Prodromal Stage

The following clinical manifestations may occur in the last weeks of pregnancy:

Shelfing

It is falling forwards of the uterine fundus making the upper abdomen looks like a shelf during standing position.

This is due to engagement of the head which brings the fetus perpendicular to the pelvic inlet in the direction of pelvic axis.

Lightening

It is the relief of upper abdominal pressure symptoms as dyspnoea, dyspepsia and palpitation due to:

– Descent in the fundal level after engagement of the head.

– Shelfing of the uterus.

Pelvic Pressure Symptoms

With engagement of the presenting part the following symptoms may occur:

– Frequency of micturition.

– Rectal tenesmus.

– Difficulty in walking.

<u>False Labor Pain (Braxton-Hicks Contractions)</u>

These are differentiated from true labor pain as follow:

- Pain is felt mainly in the abdomen.

- Irregular.

- No increase in frequency, duration and intensity.

- No effect on the cervix.

- No bulging of the membranes.

- Can be relieved by antispasmodics and sedatives.

Onset of Labor

The onset of labor is characterised by:

<u>True Labor Pain</u>

These are differentiated from false labor pain as follow:

- Pain is felt in the abdomen and radiating to the back.

- Regular.

- Progressive increase in frequency, duration and intensity (3 contractions every 10 minutes, each lasts 50-60 seconds in active phase).

- Progressive dilatation and effacement of the cervix.

- Membranes are bulging during contractions.

- Not relieved by antispasmodics or sedatives.

<u>The Show</u>

It is an expelled cervical mucus plug tinged with blood from ruptured small vessels as a result of separation of the membranes from the lower uterine segment.

Labor usually starts several hours to few days after show.

<u>Dilatation of the Cervix</u>

A closed cervix is a reliable sign that labor has not begun.

In multigravida the cervix may admit the tip of the finger before onset of labor.

<u>Formation of Bag of Forewater</u>

It bulges through the cervix and becomes tense during uterine contractions.

First Stage of Labor

History

<u>Past Obstetric History</u> in detailes.

<u>History of Present Pregnancy</u>

　Duration of pregnancy.

– Review of the patient's prenatal care.

– Medical disorders during this pregnancy.

– Complications during this pregnancy as antepartum hemorrhage.

<u>History of Present Labor</u>

– Labor pains: onset, frequency and duration.

– Passage of "show", fluid or blood per vaginum.

– Sensation of fetal movement.

Examination

<u>General Examination</u>

– Height and built.

– Maternal vital signs: pulse, temperature and blood pressure.

– Chest and heart examination.

– Lower limbs for oedema.

<u>Abdominal Examination (Leopold Maneuvers)</u>

– Fundal grip.

– Umbilical grip.

– First pelvic grip.

– Second pelvic grip.

– Fundal level.

– FHS.

– Scar of previous operations (e.g. C.S., myomectomy).

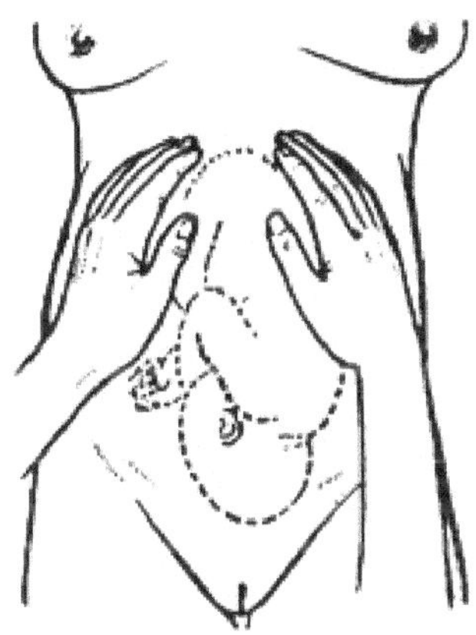

(1) Fundal Grip

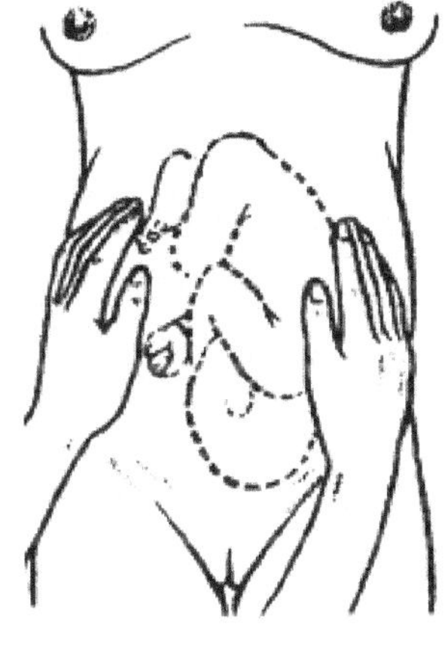

(2) Umbilical Grip

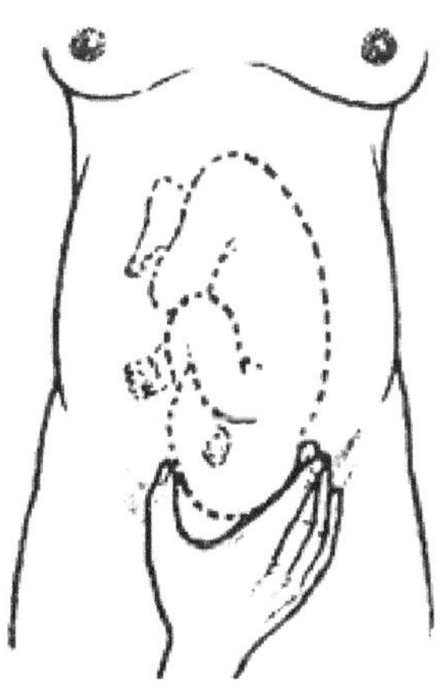

(3) First Pelvic Grip

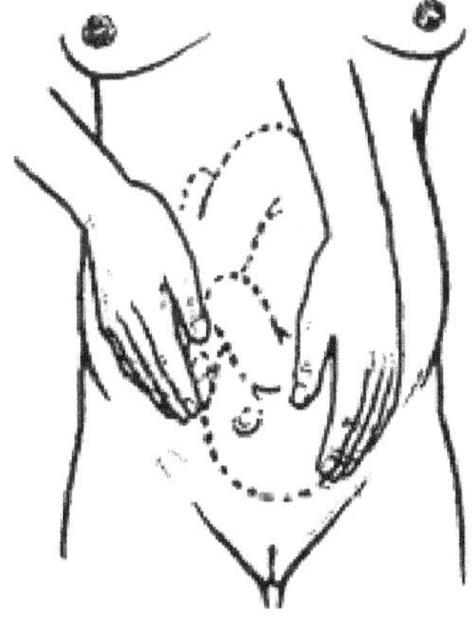

(4) Second Pelvic Grip

Abdominal Examination (Leopold Maneuvers)

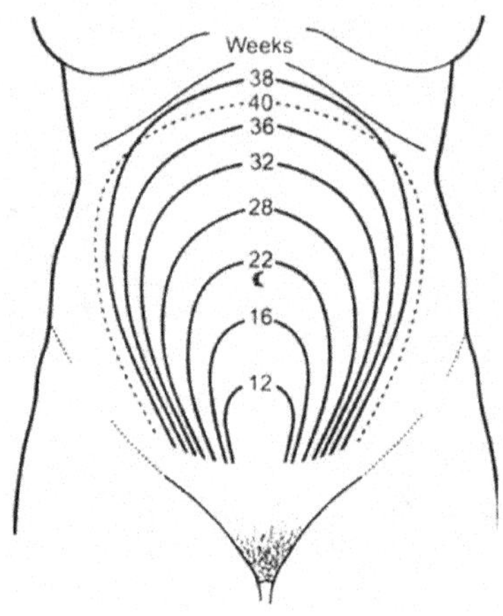

Fundal Level

Pelvic Examination

Pelvic examination is often performed using sterile gloves to decrease the risk of infection.

If membrane rupture is suspected, examination with a sterile speculum is performed to confirm pooling of amniotic fluid in the posterior fornix.

The examiner also looks for fern on a dried sample of the vaginal fluid under a microscope and checks the pH of the fluid by using a nitrazine stick or litmus paper, which turns blue if the amniotic fluid is alkalotic.

If frank bleeding is present, pelvic examination should be deferred until placenta previa is excluded with ultrasonography.

Furthermore, the pattern of contraction and the patient's presenting history may provide clues about placental abruption.

Digital examination of the cervix determines the following:

– Cervical dilatation, which ranges from 0 cm (closed or fingertip) to 10 cm (complete or fully dilated).

– Cervical effacement (assessment of the cervical length).

– Cervical position (anterior or posterior).

– Cervical consistency (soft or firm).

Palpation of the presenting part of the fetus allows the examiner to establish its station, by quantifying the distance of the body (-5 to +5 cm) that is presenting relative to the maternal ischial spines, where 0 station is in line with the plane of the maternal ischial spines).

The pelvic planes include the following:

– Pelvic inlet:

The obstetrical conjugate is the distance between the sacral promontory and the inner pubic arch; it should measure 11.5 cm or more.

The diagonal conjugate is the distance from the undersurface of the pubic arch to sacral promontory.

It is 2 cm longer than the obstetrical conjugate.

The transverse diameter of the pelvic inlet measures 13.5 cm.

– Midpelvis:

The midpelvis is the distance between the bony points of ischial spines, and it typically exceeds 12 cm.

– Pelvic outlet:

The pelvic outlet is the distance between the ischial tuberosities and the pubic arch, and usually exceeds 10 cm.

The shape of the mother's pelvis can also be assessed and classified into 4 broad categories: gynecoid, anthropoid, android, and platypelloid.

Although the gynecoid and anthropoid pelvic shapes are thought to be most favorable for vaginal delivery, many women can be classified into 1 or more pelvic types, and such distinctions can be arbitrary.

Investigations

If not done before or if indicated:

– Complete blood cell (CBC) count.

– Blood group, Rh typing.

– Urine for albumin and sugar.

– Ultrasonography.

Workup

Evacuation of the Rectum

By enema to:

– Avoid uterine inertia.

– Help the descent of the presenting part.

– Avoid contamination by faeces during delivery.

Evacuation of the Bladder

Ask the patient to micturate every 2-3 hours.

If she can not, use a catheter.

It prevents uterine inertia.

It also helps descent of the presenting part.

Preparation of the Vulva

Shave the vulva, and clean it with soap and warm water from above downwards.

Swab it with antiseptic lotion, and apply a sterile pad.

Nutrition

When labor is established no oral feeding is allowed, but sips of water.

If labor is delayed more than 8 hours, IV drip of glucose 5% or saline-glucose solution is given.

Posture

Patient is allowed to walk during the early first stage particularly with intact membranes.

If rest is needed the patient lies on her left lateral position to prevent inferior vena cava compression and hence placental insufficiency.

Patient should not bear down during the first stage as this is useless, exhausts the patient and predisposes to genital prolapse.

Pain Control

Ideal pain releif should: provide good analgesia, and be safe for the mother and fetus, and in the same time reversible if necessary.

Agents given in intermittent doses for systemic pain control include the following:

– Meperidine, 25-50 mg IV / 1-2 hours or 50-100 mg IM / 2-4 hours.

– Fentanyl, 50-100 mcg IV / hour.

– Nalbuphine, 10 mg IV or IM / 3 hours.

– Butorphanol, 1-2 mg IV or IM / 4 hours.

– Morphine, 2-5 mg IV or 10 mg IM / 4 hours.

As an alternative, regional anesthesia may be given including the following:

– Epidural:

  It provides the most effective pain relief.

  A plastic catheter is introduced into the epidural space through a needle with a curved tip.

  Intermittent doses of a local anaesthetic are injected through the catheter.

– Spinal.

– Combined spinal-epidural.

The Partogram

The frequency and strength of uterine contractions and changes in cervix and in the fetus' station and position should be assessed periodically to evaluate the progression of labor.

Although progression must be monitored, vaginal examinations should be performed only when necessary to minimize the risk of chorioamnionitis, particularly in women whose amniotic membrane has ruptured.

Partogram is the graphic recording of the course of labor including the following observations:

– Pulse every 30 minutes.

– Blood pressure every 2 hours.

– Temperature every 4 hours.

– Uterine contractions: frequency, strength and duration every 30 minutes by manual palpation or better by tocography if available.

– FHR monitoring every 15 minutes, particularly during and immediately after uterine contractions.

– Cervical dilatation.

– Descent of the presenting part.

– Degree of moulding.

– Fluid input and output.

– Drugs including oxytocins.

Name ___________________________________

Time of admission ___________________________ Date ___________________

Pains _________________ Show _________________ Ruptured membranes _________

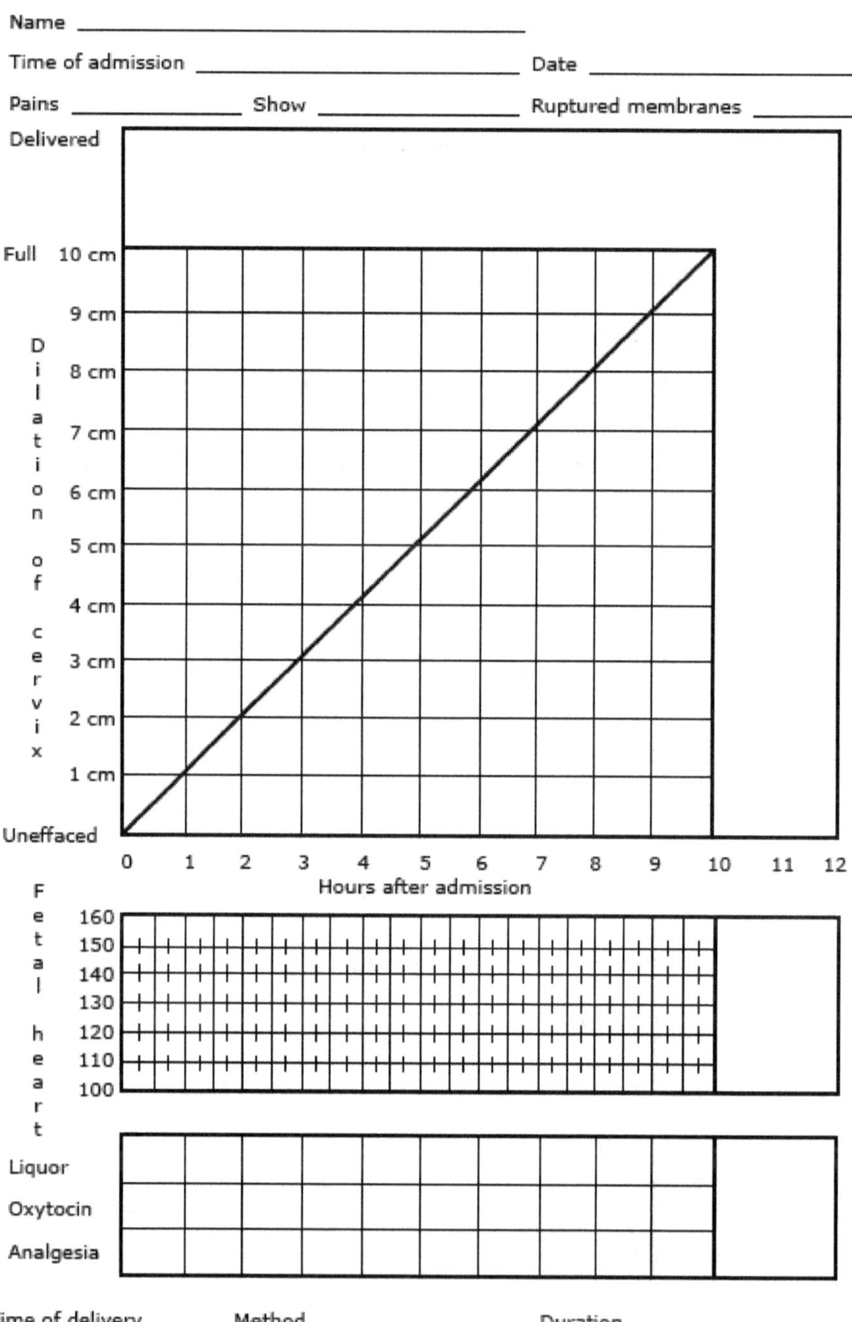

Time of delivery _______ Method _________________ Duration _________________

Partogram

Cardiotocography (CTG)

Is more valuable for continuous monitoring of both uterine contractions and FHR particularly in high risk pregnancy.

Cardiotography during labor is associated with a reduction in neonatal seizures but not cerebral palsy or infant mortality; however, continuous monitoring is associated with increased cesarean and operative vaginal deliveries.

If nonreassuring fetal heart rate tracings by cardiotography (eg, late decelerations) are noted, a fetal scalp electrode may be applied to generate sensitive readings of beat-to-beat variability.

A framework has been suggested to classify and standardize the interpretation of a fetal heart rate monitoring pattern according to the risk of fetal acidemia with the intention of minimizing neonatal acidemia without excessive obstetric intervention.

The existing data provide limited support for the use of fetal pulse oximetry when used in the presence of a nonreassuring fetal heart rate tracing to reduce cesarean delivery for nonreassuring fetal status.

Further evaluation of a fetus at risk for labor intolerance or distress can be accomplished with blood sampling from fetal scalp capillaries.

This procedure allows for a direct assessment of fetal oxygenation and blood pH.

A pH of < 7.20 warrants further investigation for the fetus' well-being and for possible resuscitation or surgical intervention.

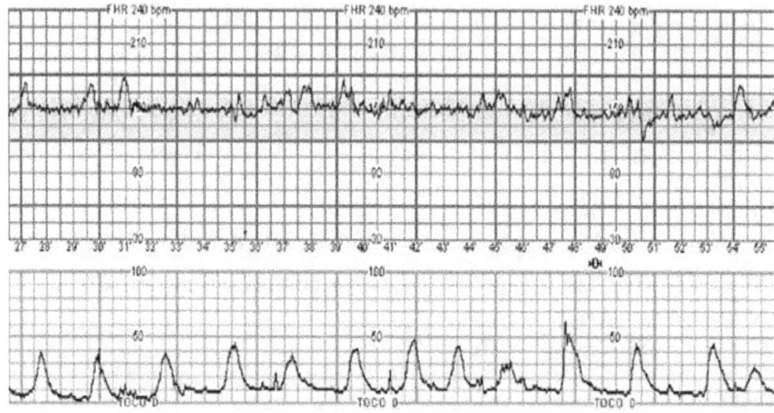

Cardiotocography (CTG)

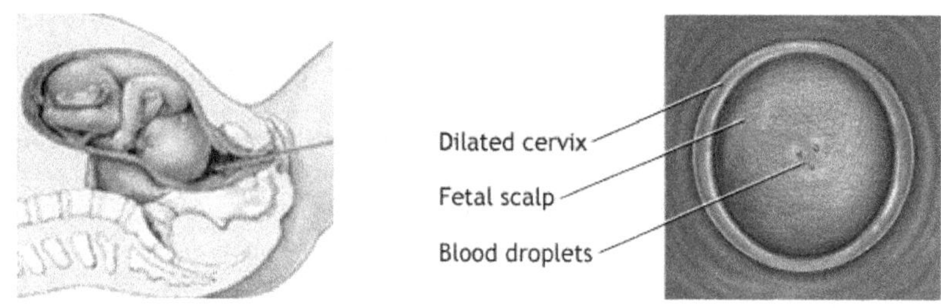

Fetal Scalp pH Testing

<u>Augmention of Labor</u>

Two methods of augmenting labor have been established.

The traditional method involves the use of low doses of oxytocin with long intervals between dose increments.

For example, low-dose infusion of oxytocin is started at 1 mili IU/min and increased by 1-2 mili IU/min every 20-30 minutes until adequate uterine contraction is obtained.

The second method, or active management of labor, involves a protocol of clinical management that aims to optimize uterine contractions and shorten labor.

This protocol includes strict criteria for admission to the labor and delivery unit, early amniotomy, hourly cervical examinations, early diagnosis of inefficient uterine activity (if the cervical dilation rate is < 1.0 cm/h), and high-dose oxytocin infusion if uterine activity is inefficient.

Oxytocin infusion starts at 4 mili IU/min (or even 6 mili IU/min) and increases by 4 mili IU/min (or 6 mili IU/min) every 15 minutes until a rate of 7 contractions per 15 minutes is achieved or until the maximum infusion rate of 36 mili IU/min is reached.

SECOND STAGE OF LABOR

It is the stage of expulsion of the fetus.

Begins with full cervical dilatation.

Ends with the delivery of the fetus.

Its duration is about 1 hour in primigravida and 30 minutes in multipara.

MECHANISM

The ability of the fetus to successfully negotiate the pelvis during labor involves changes in position of its head during its passage in labor.

The mechanisms of labor, also known as the cardinal movements, are described in relation to a vertex presentation, as is the case in 95% of all pregnancies.

Although labor and delivery occurs in a continuous fashion, the cardinal movements of labor are described as discrete sequences, as discussed below.

Engagement

The widest diameter of the presenting part (with a well-flexed head, where the largest transverse diameter of the fetal occiput is the biparietal diameter) enters the maternal pelvis in the oblique or transverse diameter of the pelvic inlet.

On the pelvic examination, the presenting part is at 0 station, or at the level of the maternal ischial spines.

Descent

The downward passage of the presenting part through the pelvis.

It is continuous throughout labor particularly during the second stage and caused by:

- Uterine contractions and retractions.

- The auxiliary forces which is bearing down brought by contraction of the diaphragm and abdominal muscles.

- The unfolding of the fetus i.e. straightening of its body due to contractions of the circular muscles of the uterus.

Flexion

As the fetal vertex descents, it encounters resistance from the bony pelvis or the soft tissues of the pelvic floor, resulting in passive flexion of the fetal occiput.

The suboccipito-bregmatic diameter (9.5 cm) passes through the birth canal instead of the suboccipito-frontal diameter (10 cm).

Internal Rotation

As the head descends, the occiputis rotated about 45° in the direction of levator ani muscles i.e. downwards, forwards and inwards.

It occurs at the level of the plane of the greatest pelvic dimension.

Internal rotation brings the anteroposterior diameter of the head in line with the anteroposterior diameter of the pelvic outlet.

Extension

With further descent and full flexion of the head, the base of the occiput comes in contact with the inferior margin of the pubic symphysis.

Upward resistance from the pelvic floor and downward forces from the uterine contractions cause the occiput to extend around the symphysis.

This is followed by the delivery of the fetus' head.

Restitution

When the fetus' head is free of resistance, it untwists about 45° left or right, returning to its original anatomic position in relation to the body (undo the twist of the neck caused by internal rotation).

External Rotation

The shoulders enter the pelvis in the opposite oblique diameter to that previously passed by the head.

When the anterior shoulder meets the pelvic floor it rotates anteriorly 45°.

This movement is transmitted to the head so it rotates 45°in the same direction of restitution.

Expulsion

After the fetus' head is delivered, further descent brings the anterior shoulder to the level of the pubic symphysis.

The posterior shoulder is delivered first by lateral flexion of the spine.

The anterior shoulder then follows, then the rest of the body.

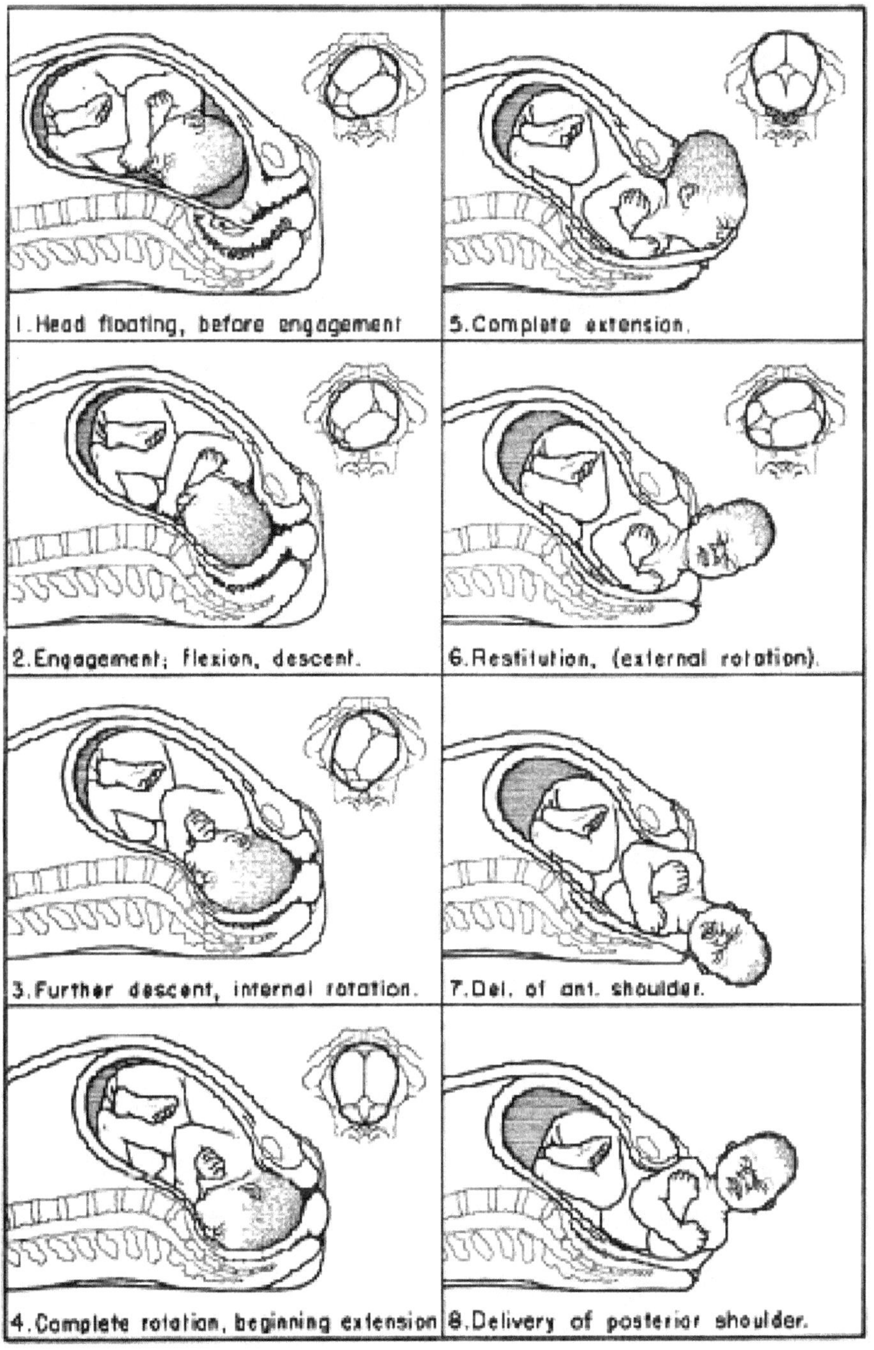

Cardinal Movements of Labor

MANAGEMENT

When the woman enters the second stage of labor with complete cervical dilatation, the fetal heart rate should be monitored or auscultated at least every 5 minutes and after each contraction during the second stage.

Although the parturient may be encouraged to push in concordance with the contractions during the second stage, many women with epidural anesthesia who do not feel the urge to push may allow the fetus to descend passively, with a period of rest before active pushing begins.

When a prolonged second stage of labor is encountered, assessment of the parturient, the fetus, and the expulsive forces is warranted.

When second-stage arrest is diagnosed, the clinician has several management options (expectant management, operative vaginal delivery by forceps or vacuum, or cesarean delivery).

Delivery of the Fetus

When delivery is imminent, the mother is usually positioned supine with her knees bent (ie, dorsal lithotomy position), though delivery can occur with the mother in any position, including the lateral (Sims) position, the partial sitting or squatting position, or on her hands and knees.

The lower abdomen, upper parts of the thighs, vulva and perineum are swabbed with antiseptic lotion.

Sterile legs and towels are applied.

Ask the patient to bear down during contractions and relax in between.

Delivery of the Head

Crowning is the word used to describe when the fetal head forcibly extends the vaginal outlet.

Episiotomy is done if indicated.

Ritgen maneuver can be performed to deliver the head.

Draped with a sterile towel, the heel of the clinician's hand is placed over the posterior perineum overlying the fetal chin, and pressure is applied upward to extend the fetus' head.

The other hand is placed over the fetus' occiput, with pressure applied downward to flex its head.

Thus, the head is held in mid position until it is delivered, followed by suctioning of the oropharynx and nares.

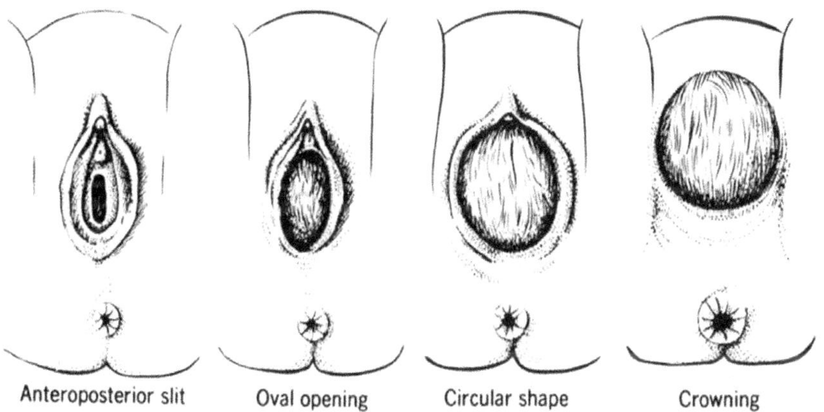

Crowning

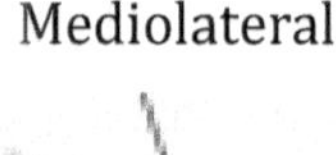

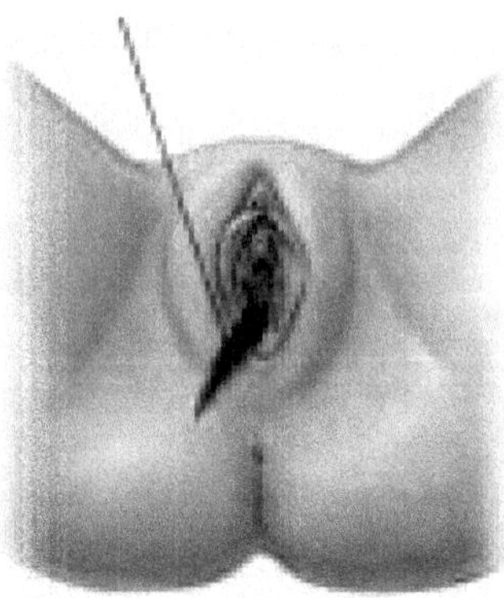

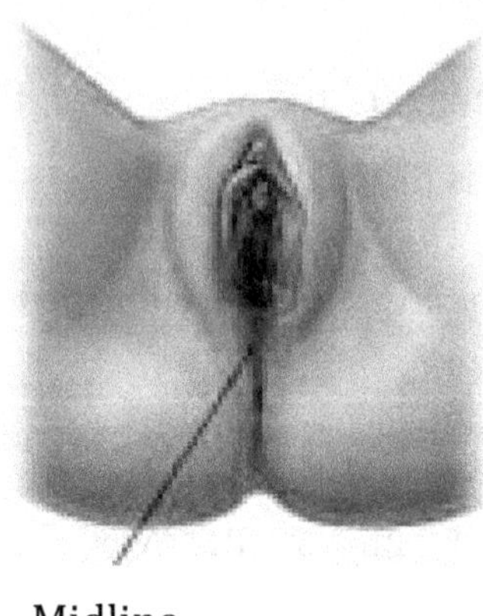

Episiotomy

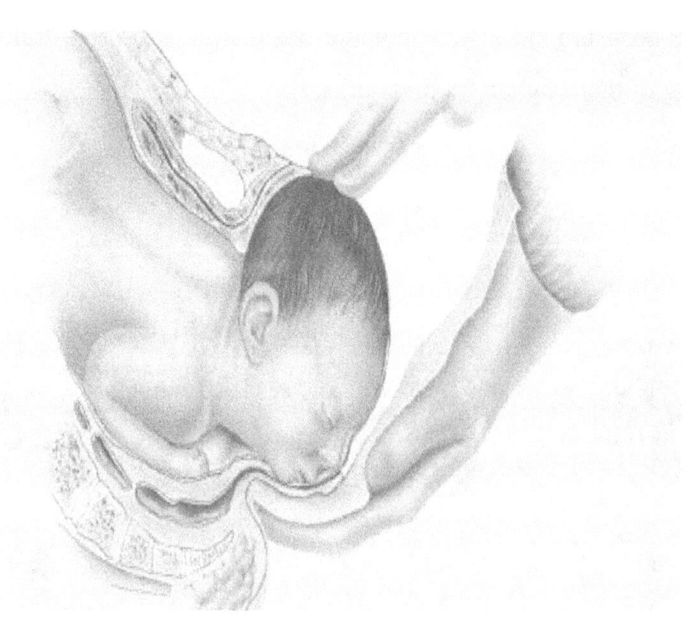

Ritgen Maneuver

<u>Delivery of the Shoulders</u>

Gentle downward traction is applied to the head till the anterior shoulder slips under the symphysis pubis.

The head is lifted upwards to deliver the posterior shoulder first then downwards to deliver the anterior shoulder.

Of note, some providers, in an attempt to avoid shoulder dystocia, deliver the anterior shoulder prior to restitution of the fetal head.

<u>Delivery of the Body</u>

Usually slips without difficulty otherwise gentle traction is applied to complete delivery.

Clamping the Cord

The baby is held by its ankles with the head downwards at a lower level than its mother for few seconds.

This is contraindicated in preterm babies, erythroblastosis fetalis, and suspicion of intracranial hemorrhage.

This may be enhanced by milking the cord towards the baby, to add about 100 ml of blood to its circulation.

The cord is divided between 2 clamps to avoid bleeding from a possible second uniovular twin.

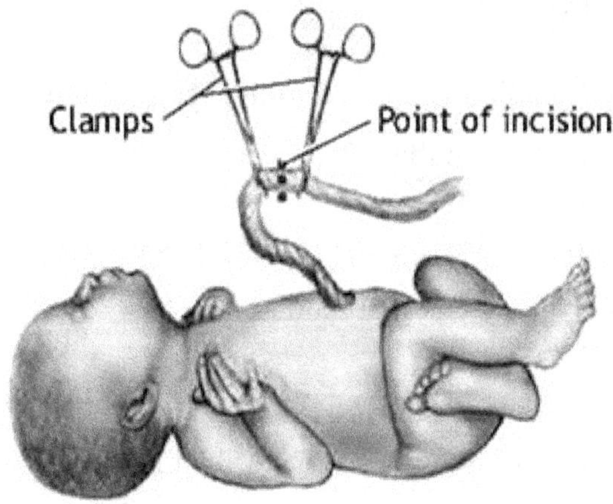

Clamping the Cord

<u>THIRD STAGE OF LABOR</u>

It is the stage of expulsion of the placenta and membranes.

Begins after delivery of the fetus.

Ends with expulsion of the placenta and membranes.

Its duration is about 10-20 minutes in both primi and multipara.

<u>MECHANISM</u>

The third stage is composed of 3 phases: placental separation, descent, and expulsion.

After delivery of the fetus, the uterus continues to contract and retract.

As the placenta is inelastic, it starts to separate through the spongiosa layer by one of the following mechanisms:

<u>Schultze's Mechanism (80%)</u>

The central area of the placenta separates first and placenta is delivered like an inverted umbrella.

There is less blood loss and less liability for retention of fragments.

<u>Duncan's Mechanism (20%)</u>

The lower edge of the placenta separates first and placenta is delivered side ways.

There is more liability of bleeding and retained fragments.

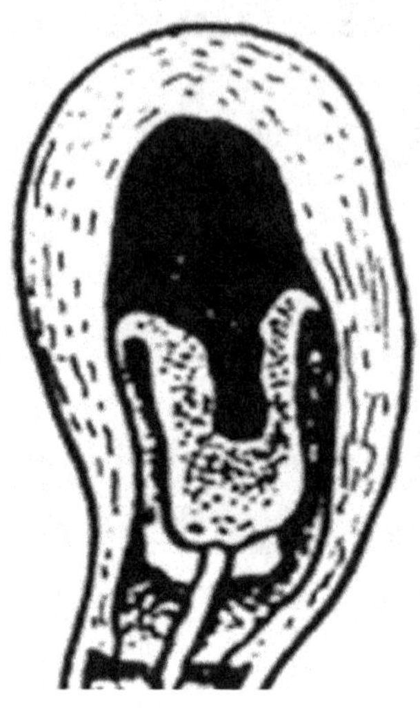

Schultze's Mechanism

Duncan's Mechanism

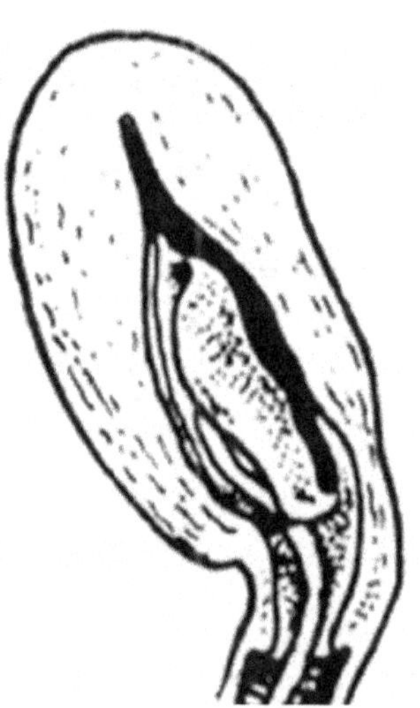

Mechanism of Placental Delivery

MANAGEMENT

Delivery of Placenta

Conservative (Expectant) Method

Put the ulnar border of the left hand just above the fundus at the level of the umbilicus to detect any bleeding inside the uterus known by rising level of the atonic uterus.

Wait for signs of placental separation and descent but do not massage the uterus.

<u>Signs of Placental Separation and Descent</u>

- The body of the uterus becomes smaller, harder and globular.

- The fundal level rises as the upper segment overrides the lower uterine segment which is now distended with the placenta.

- Suprapubic bulge due to presence of the placenta in the lower uterine segment.

- Elongation of the cord particularly on pressing on the uterine fundus and it does not recede back into the vagina on relieving the pressure.

- Gush of blood from the vagina.

As soon as these signs are detected massage the uterus to induce its contraction.

Ask the patient to bear down and push the uterus downwards to deliver the placenta.

Hold the placenta between the two hands and roll it to make the membranes like a rope in order not to miss a part of it.

Give ergometrine 0.5 mg or oxytocin 5 units IM after delivery of the placenta to help uterine contraction and minimise blood loss.

These may be given before delivery of the placenta.

Active (Brandt-Andrews) Method

With delivery of the anterior shoulder, 0.5 mg ergometrine or syntometrine (0.5 mg ergometrine + 5 units oxytocin) is given IM.

When the uterus contracts, put the left hand suprapubic and push the uterus upwards while gentle downward and backward traction is applied on the cord by the right hand.

When the placenta is delivered it is rolled as in the conservative method.

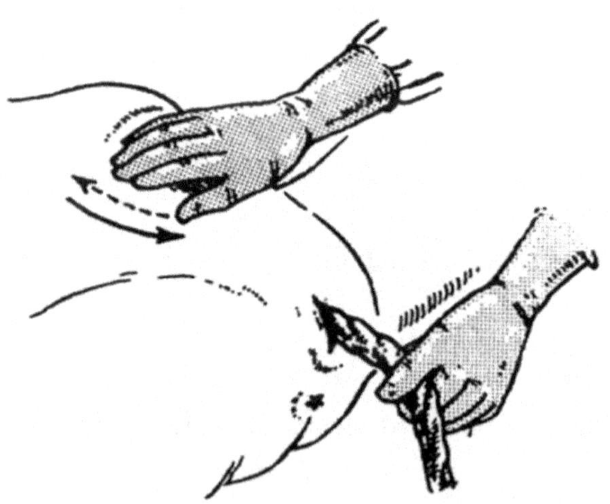

Brandt-Andrews Method

After Delivery of Placenta

Examine the placenta and membranes by exploring it on a plain surface to be sure that it is complete.

If there is missed part, exploration of the uterus is done under general anaesthesia.

Ongoing blood loss and a boggy uterus suggest uterine atony.

A thorough examination of the birth canal, including the cervix and the vagina, the perineum, and the distal rectum, is warranted, and repair of episiotomy or perineal / vaginal lacerations should be carried out.

Care of the Newborn

Clearance of Air Passages

The newborn is placed in supine position with the head lower down.

A metal, rubber or better disposable plastic catheter is used to aspirate the mucus from the pharynx and mouth directly by the physician's mouth or by attach it to an electric suction pump.

Crying of the baby is usually occurs within seconds, if delayed slapping its soles, flexion and extension of the legs and rubbing the back usually stimulate breathing.

Apgar Score

Is calculated at 1 and 5 minutes and further steps of resuscitation are arranged according to it.

Umbilical Cord

A disposable plastic umbilical clamp is applied about 5 cm from the umbilicus to avoid the possibility of tying an umbilical hernia then cut about 1.5 cm distal to the clamp.

Inspect for bleeding and paint it with alcohol.

Weight

Weight the newborn and record it.

Congenital Anomalies

The newborn is examined for injuries or congenital anomalies.

Care of Eyes

An antibiotic eye drops are instilled into the eyes as a prophylaxis against ophthalmia neonatorum.

Dressing

Dressing as well as all previous procedures should be done in a warm place better under radiant warmer to prevent heat loss which occurs rapidly after delivery increasing the metabolism and acidosis.

Identification

Identification of the baby by a plastic bracelet on which its mother's name is written.

Fourth Stage of Labor

It is the stage of early recovery.

Begins immediately after expulsion of the placenta and membranes.

Lasts for one hour.

Routine uterine massage is usually done every 15 minutes during this period.

Careful observation for the patient, particularly atony of the uterus and vaginal bleeding is essential.

ABNORMAL LABOR

MALPRESENTATIONS AND MALPOSITION

Definitions

Lie: The relationship of the long axis of the fetus to that of the mother.

It may be longitudinal, transverse or oblique.

Presentation: The portion of the fetus that is foremost or presenting in the birth canal.

Malpresentations: All presentations of the fetus other than the vertex:

−Face.

−Brow.

−Breech.

−Transverse.

−Compound.

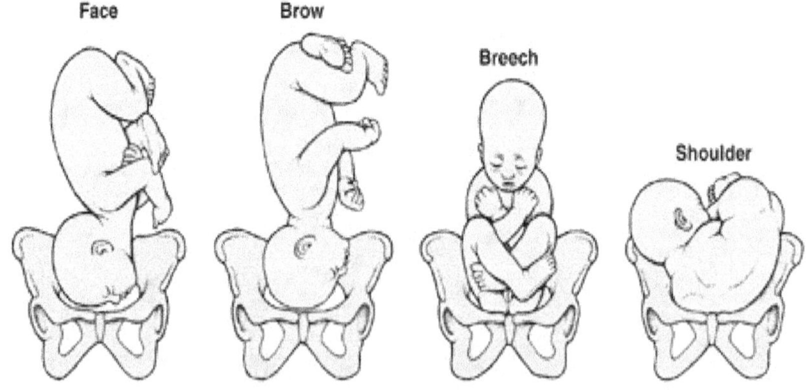

Position

Reference point on the presenting part, and how it relates to the maternal pelvis.

Normal position is occipito-anterior position (OA): when the fetal occiput is directed towards the mother's symphyisis or anteriorly.

Malposition

Occipito-posterior (OP): when the fetal occiput is directed towards the mother's sacrum or posteriorly.

Causes

−Defects of the power: laxity of the abdominal muscles, exaggerated dextrorotation of the uterus.

−Defects of passage: contracted pelvis, android pelvis, pelvic tumor, uterine anomaly, placenta previa.

−Defect of passenger: preterm fetus, macrosomia, multiple pregnancy, polyhydramnios, anacephaly and hydrocephaly, IUFD.

OCCIPITO-POSTERIOR POSITION (OP)

It is a vertex presentation in which the fetal back is directed posteriorly.

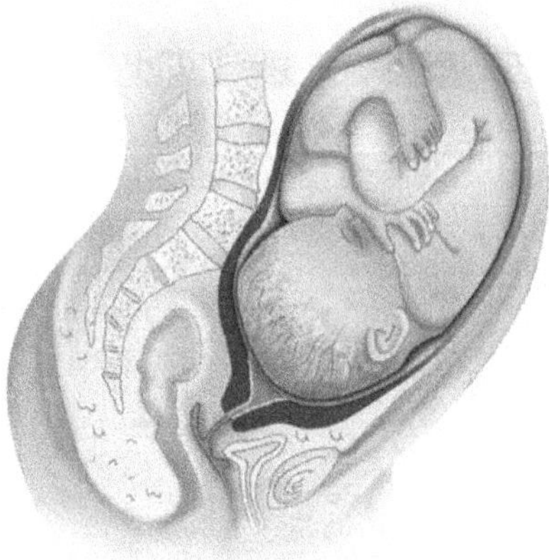

Diagnosis

Vaginal Examination

– The anterior fontanelle is palpated.

– Identify the sagittal suture which is mostly asymmetric.

– Dilation is often asymmetric, you can feel the fetal ear and a persistent anterior cervical lip is common.

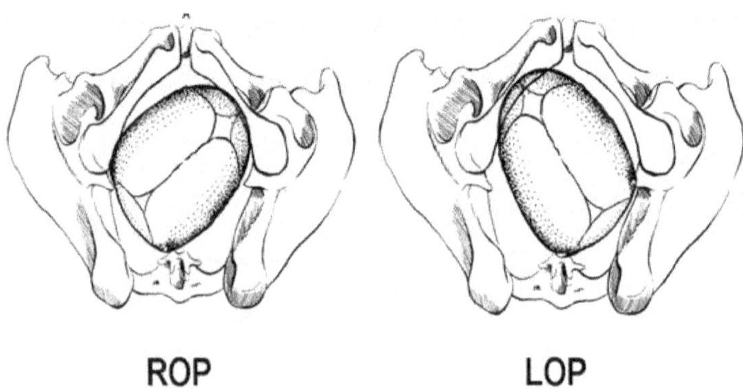

Management

−Spontaneous delivery is possible: make sure uterine contractions are adequate and no fetal distress.

−Manual rotation.

−Vacuum extraction delivery.

−CS should always be the backup method of delivery for any occipito-posterior presentation that cannot be safely delivered vaginally.

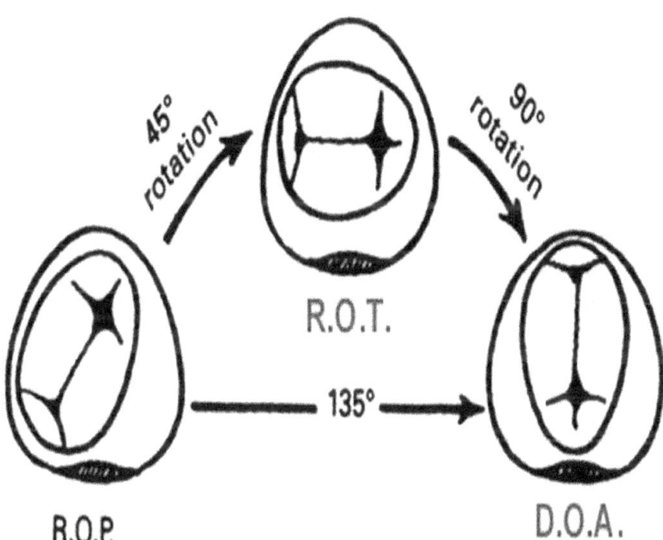

FACE PRESENTATION

Cephalic presentation in which the head is fully extended.

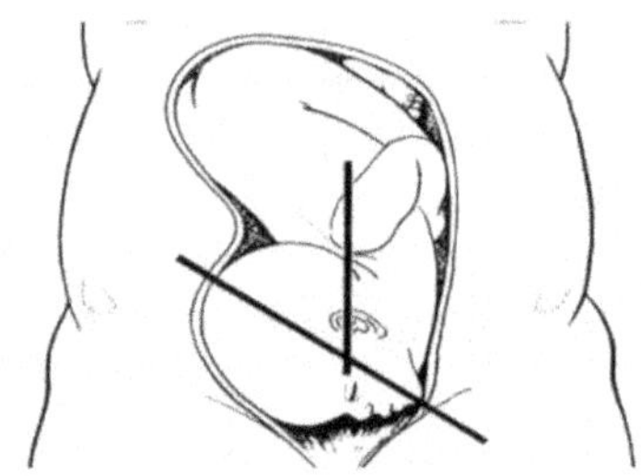

Diagnosis

Vaginal Examination

– The face is palpable and the point of reference is the chin; you should

feel the mouth and be careful not to confuse it with breech presentation.

– It is necessary to distinguish the mento-anterior position from mento-

posterior position.

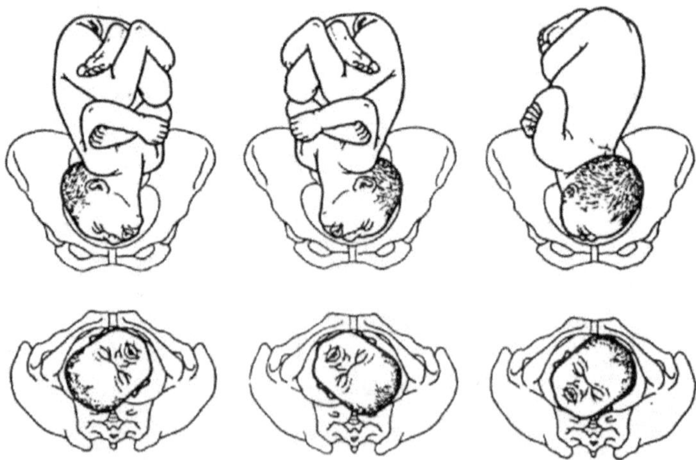

Management

Mento-anterior Position

–If the cervix is fully dilated: vaginal delivery.

–If there is slow progress and no sign of obstruction: augment labor.

–If descent is unsatisfactory: perform a CS.

Mento-posterior Position

–Deliver by CS.

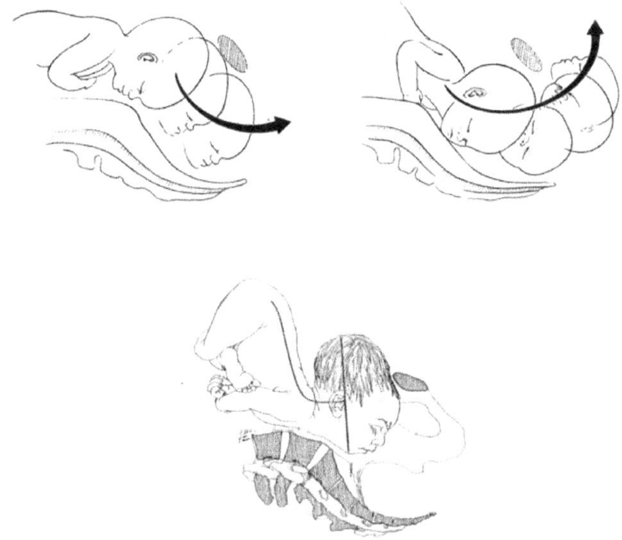

Face Presentation, direct mento-posterior vaginal delivery is impossible.

<u>BROW PRESENTATION</u>

Cephalic presentation in which the head is midway between flexion and extension.

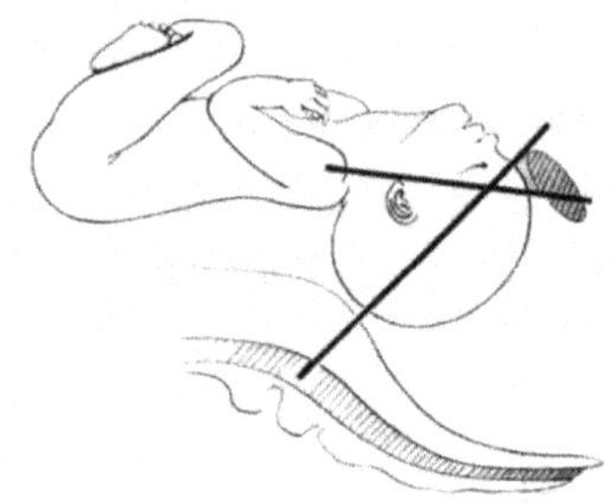

<u>Diagnosis</u>

<u>Vaginal Examination</u>

−The anterior fontannel and the orbital notches are felt; the referral point is the nasal apex.

−The chin is not felt.

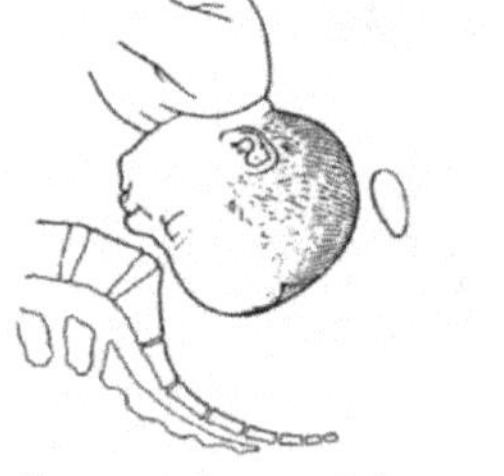

Brow posterior presentation

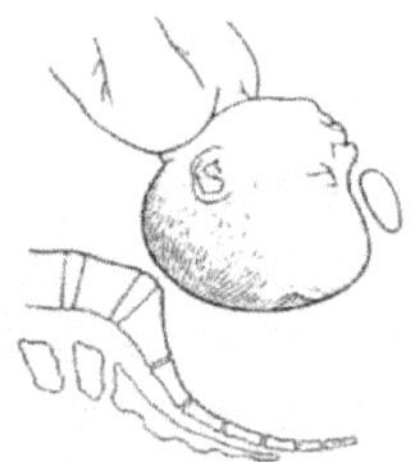

Brow anterior presentation

<u>Management</u>

−Deliver by CS.

BREECH PRESENTATION

Longitudinal lie in which the buttocks and/or the feet are the presenting part.

Types

−Complete (flexed) breech: both legs are flexed at the hips and the knees.

−Frank (extended) breech: both legs are flexed at the hips and extended at the knees.

−Footling breech: a leg is extended at the hip and the knee.

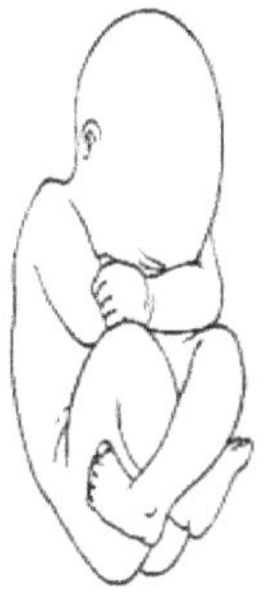 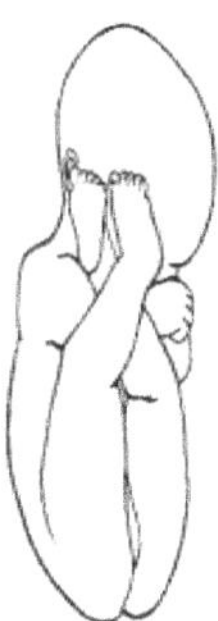 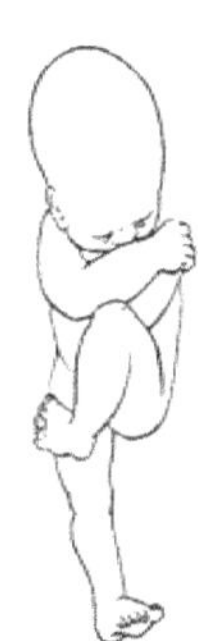

Diagnosis

Abdominal Examination

−The head is felt in the upper abdomen.

−The breech in the pelvic brim.

Vaginal Examination

−The buttocks and/or feet are felt.

−Thick dark meconium is normal.

Complications

−Entrapment of the after coming head.

−Nuchal arm.

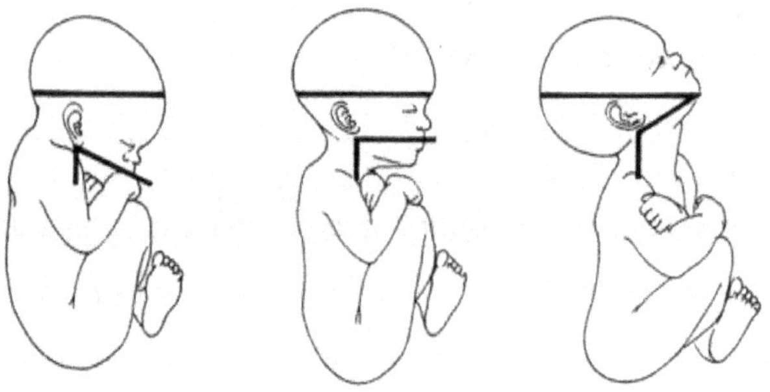

Management

External Cephalic Version

Consider at 37 weeks if all requirements are met:

−Adequate amniotic fluid.

−Placenta in fundal position.

−No uterine anomalies.

−No previous uterine scar.

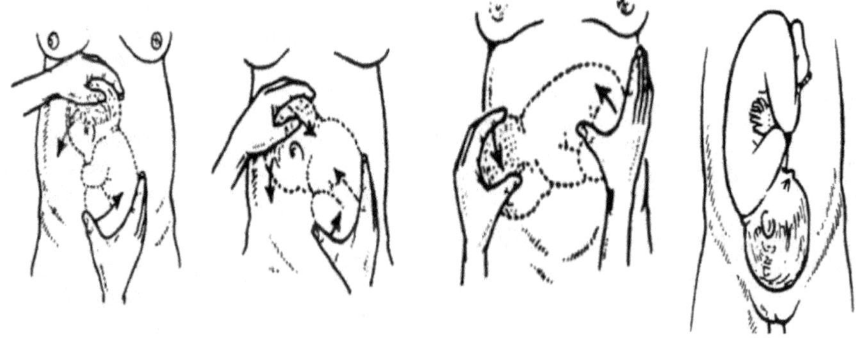

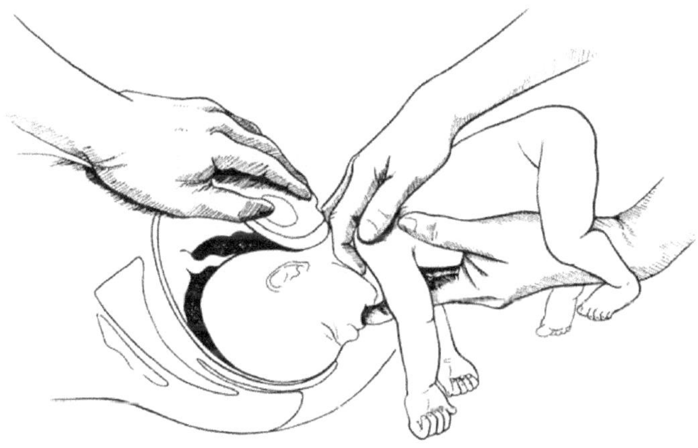

Indications for CS

−Primigravida.

−Footling breech.

−Hyperextension of fetal head.

−Nuchal arm.

−Macrosomia.

−Severe prematurity, IUGR, placental insufficiency.

−Other indications for CS.

TRANSVERSE PRESENTATION

Longitudinal axis of the fetus does not coinside with that of the mother.

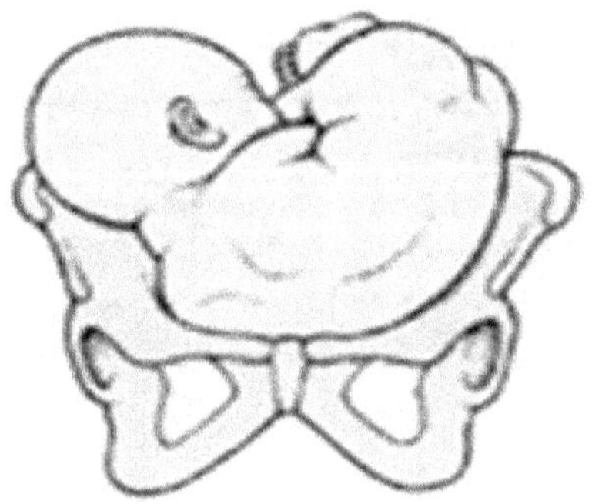

Diagnosis

During Pregnancy

− Inspection: abdomen is broader from side to side.

− Palpation: the fundus feels empty and the fundal level is lower than expected.

− Ultrasound confirms the diagnosis.

During Labor

− On vaginal examination, the scapula is felt as point of reference.

− Ultrasound confirms the diagnosis.

Management

− Deliver by CS.

CORD PRESENTATION AND PROLAPSE

Definitions

−Cord Presentation: umbilical cord lies below the presenting part with intact membranes.

−Cord Prolapse: umbilical cord lies below the presenting part with ruptured membranes.

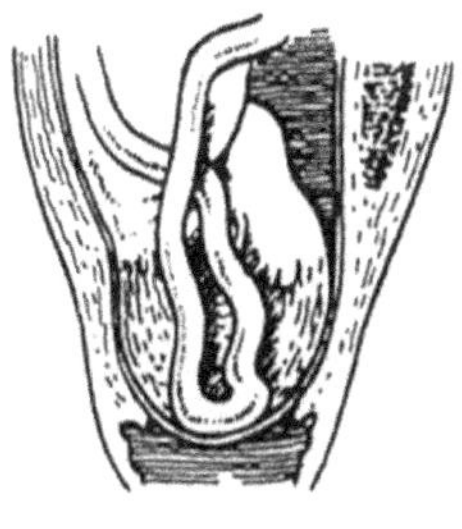

Cord Presentation
Membranes Intact

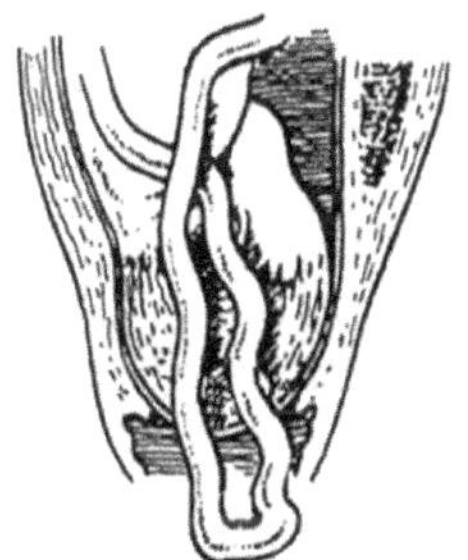

Cord Prolapse
Membranes Ruptured

Causes

−Long cord.

−Breech, shoulder, and other malpresentations.

−Contracted pelvis.

−Preterm labor +/- low birth weight <2500 g.

−Polyhydramnios.

−Multiple pregnancy (usually the second twin).

−Placenta praevia.

Diagnosis

−Feeling of a soft usually pulsatile structure on vaginal examination.

−Fetal distress.

Management

Pulsating Cord

−Delivery by CS is the safest method.

−Rarely, with a fully dilated cervix, deliver the head immediately by the forceps or the vacuum extractor.

Non-pulsating Cord

−If the foetus is certainly dead, labor is left to continue until eventual vaginal delivery.

MULTIPLE PREGNANCY

Definition

More than one fetus in the uterus.

Mostly twin pregnancy but others may be encountered, triplets or plus.

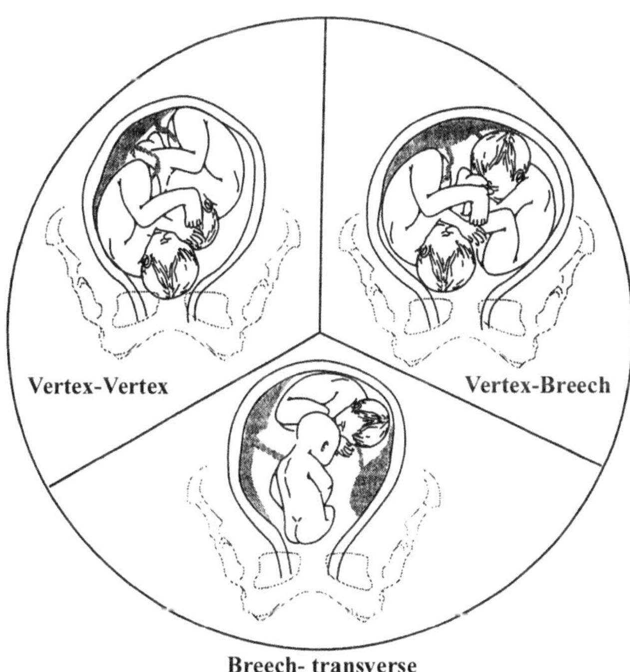

Causes

−Ovulation induction.

−Assisted reproductive techniques.

−Hereditary factors.

−Previous multiple pregnancy.

Diagnosis

−Exaggerated symptoms of pregnancy.

−Fundal height larger the gestational age.

−Two audible fetal heart beats.

−Multiple fetal parts or more than two fetal poles.

Investigations

−Ultrasound to determine chorionicity.

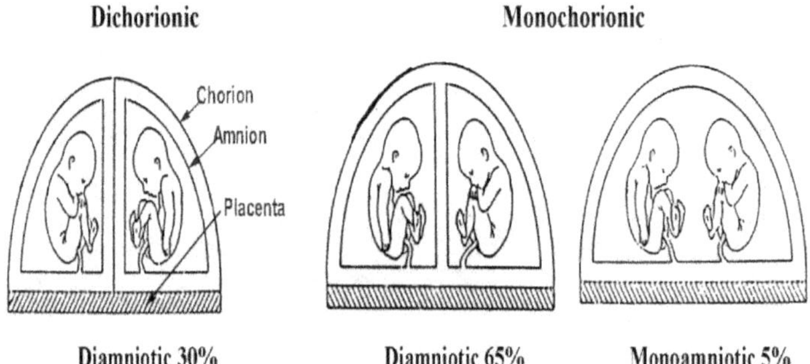

Complications

−Increased risk of miscarriage.

−Prematurity.

−Intrauterine fetal growth retardation.

−Fetal transfusion syndrome (twin-twin transfusion syndrome).

−Malpresentations.

−Pregnancy induced diabetes.

−Pregnancy induced hypertension.

−Antepartum hemorrhage.

−Postpartum hemorrhage.

−Polyhydramnios.

−Premature rupture of membranes.

Management

<u>Antenatal</u>

−Bed rest.

−Increase nutrition.

−Routine antenatal care.

−Ultrasound to determine presentation of first twin, detect anomalies.

−Monitor for associated obstetric complications.

<u>Vaginal Delivery</u>

−The first twin is cephalic.

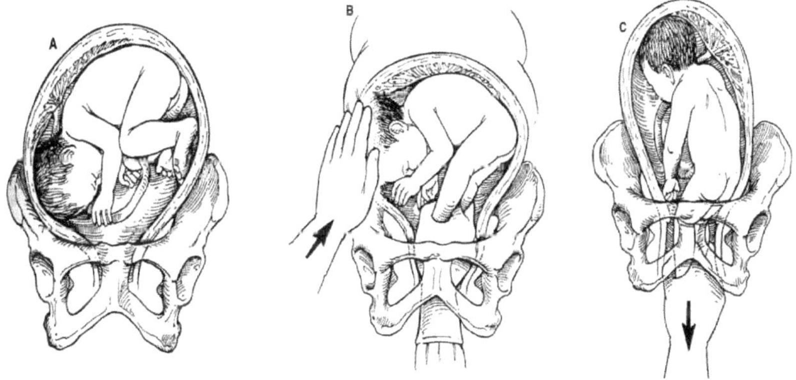

Delivery of the second twin (transverse lie) by Internal podalic version (IPV) and vaginal breech extraction

<u>Cesarean Section</u>

−The first twin is not cephalic (locked twin).

−Retained living second twin.

−More than two fetuses.

−Previous uterine scar.

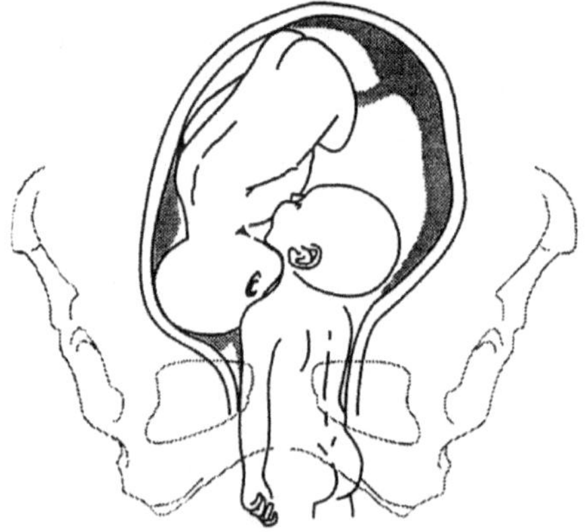

Locked Twin

<u>Third stage</u>

−Look for and anticipate postpartum hemorrhage.

<u>LABOR DYSTOCIA</u>

<u>Definition</u>

Dystocia of labor is defined as difficult labor or abnormally slow progress of labor.

<u>Causes</u>

−Power (inadequate uterine contractions, contraction ring of the uterus, myomas, uterine scar).

−Passage (abnormal pelvic anatomy).

−Passenger (macrosomia, malpresentation, malposition, fetal anomalies).

<u>Diagnosis</u>

−Lumbar and abnormal back pain due to ineffective contractions.

−Dehydration.

−Anxiety.

−Maternal exhaustion.

−Bandl's ring

−Fetal distress.

−Failure of cervix to dilate despite good uterine contractions.

−Edema of the cervix and vulva.

−Failure of the fetal head to descend.

−Arrested labor.

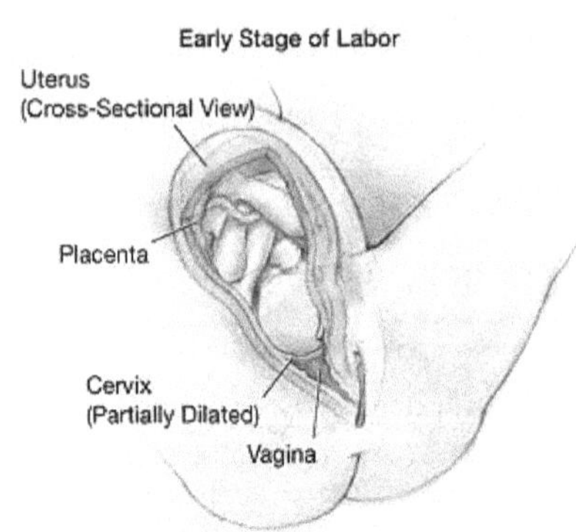

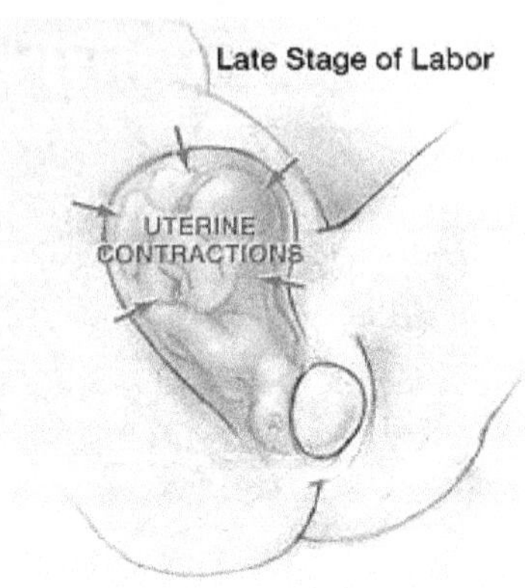

Obstructed Labor

Investigations

−Fetal monitoring with a partogram and CTG.

−Ultrasonography.

Complications

−Fetal distress.

−Fetal hypoxia / asphyxia.

−Fetal death.

−Rupture of the uterus.

−Birth canal injuries (cervical tears, vaginal and perineal lacerations).

−PPH.

−Postpartum endometritis.

−Maternal death.

Management

– Evaluation of uterine power, pelvis, passenger, pain.

– Fetal monitoring.

– Correction of malposition: occipito-posterior position is significant contributor to dystocia; can be corrected by spontaneous rotation, manual rotation or by vacuum / forceps.

– Active management:

Pattern	Primi	Multi	Management
Prolonged latent phase	>20h	>14h	Amniotomy, Prostaglandins or oxytocin
Active phase, arrest of dilation	≤1.2cm/h	≤1.5cm/h	Amniotomy or oxytocin, If no success – CS
No cervical dilation	≥2h	≥2h	Amniotomy or oxytocin, If no success – CS
Arrest of descent in second stage	≥1h	≥1h	Amniotomy or oxytocin, If no success – CS

<u>SHOULDER DYSTOCIA</u>

<u>Definition</u>

The fetal shoulders fail to deliver shortly after the fetal head.

<u>Causes</u>

–Fetal macrosomia.

–Diabetes.

–Maternal obesity.

–Short in stature.

–Age >35.

–Abnormal pelvis.

–Postterm pregnancy.

<u>Diagnosis</u>

–A prolonged first or second stage of labor.

–Turtle sign: appearance and retraction of the fetal head.

–Head bobbing in the second stage.

–Failure to restitute.

–No shoulder rotation or descent.

<u>Complications</u>

–Fetal injury (such as brachial plexus injury) and fetal death.

–Maternal injuries and postpartum hemorrhage.

Management

−Ask for help of an obstetrician, for anesthesia, and for pediatrics.

−Episiotomy.

−McRoberts' maneuver: hyperflexing the mother's legs tightly to her abdomen +/- suprapubic pressure.

−Rubin maneuver or posterior pressure on the anterior shoulder, which would bring the fetus in an oblique position.

−Woods' screw maneuver which leads to turning the anterior shoulder to the posterior and vice versa.

−Manual delivery of posterior arm.

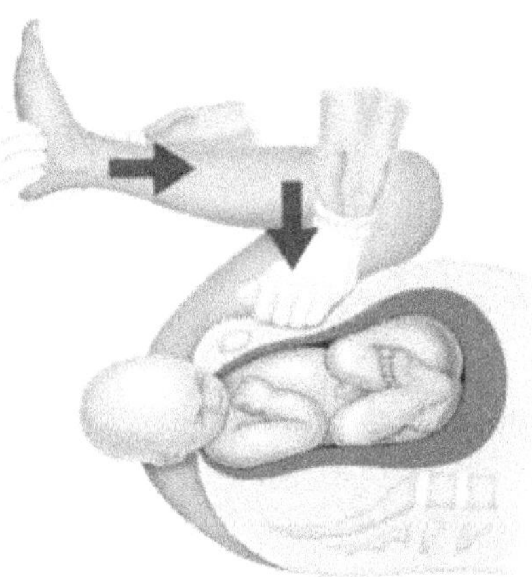

McRoberts' Maneuver

UTERINE RUPTURE

Definition

Uterine rupture refers to a tear or separation of the uterine wall.

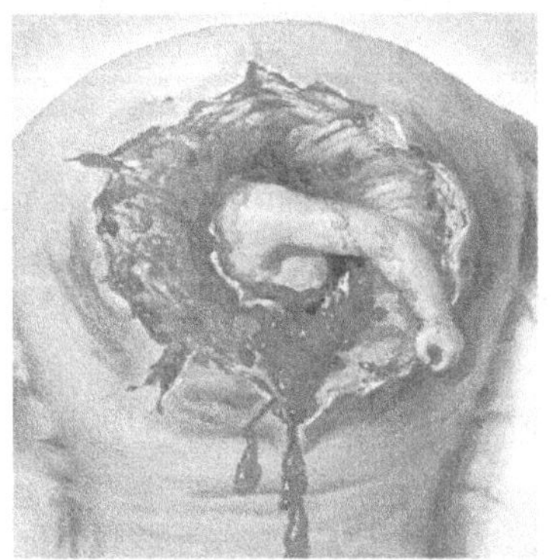

Causes

−Multiparity.

−Previous uterine scar.

−Malpresentation and malposition.

−Misuse of uterotonics.

−Placenta insertion anomalies.

−Contracted pelvis.

−Obstructed labor.

−Uterine manoeuvers.

−Instrumental deliveries.

−Trial of labor after CS.

Diagnosis

−Pre-rupture bandle ring sign.

−Sudden, severe abdominal pain (may decrease after rupture).

−Bleeding – intra-abdominal and/or vaginal.

−Cessation of uterine contractions.

−Tender abdomen.

−Absent fetal heart activity.

−Easily palpable fetal parts on the abdomen.

−Rapid maternal pulse.

−Hypovolaemic shock most of the time.

Investigations

−Full blood Count and blood group crossmatch.

−Clotting profile.

−CTG monitoring.

−Ultrasound in a stable patient (In cases of uterine dehiscence suspicion).

Complications

Fetal demise.

−Uterine multi-laceration leading to Hysterectomy.

−Bladder laceration.

−Maternal death.

Management

Management of Shock

−Senior obstetrician, pediatrician and anaesthetist for assistance.

−Assess for clinical signs of shock e.g. cool, clammy, pale, rapid pulse, decreased blood pressure.

−Insert 2 large intravenous accesses using 14-16 gauge cannulas with appropriate intravenous fluid.

−Order 2-4 units of packed red cells.

−Administer oxygen via face mask 6L/min.

−Ensure the woman remains with her legs bent or in lithotomy to perfuse the brain.

Emergency Laparotomy

−Conservative or hysterectomy and repair complications (bladder or ureter tear…).

−If conservative, contraception for at least 2 years.

−Elective CS for the next pregnancy at 39 weeks of gestation or if uterine contractions start.

CERVICAL TEARS

Causes

−Improper use of oxytocin and /or prostaglandins.

−Faulty application of forceps or ventouse.

−After coming head in breech presentation.

−Obstructed labor.

−Some cases of precipitate labor.

−Previous cervical cerclage.

−Placenta previa.

Complications

−PPH.

−Extension of the tear upwards into the lower segment or broad ligament.

−Infections.

−Incompetent cervix.

Management

−Management of shock.

−Suturing should start above the apex of cervical tear.

PERINEAL TEARS

Definition

Tears of the perineal tissue between the vagina and rectum.

Grades

−1st degree injury to perineal skin.

−2nd degree injury involving perineal muscles but not the anal sphincter.

−3rd degree involvement is of the anal sphincter.

−4th degree involvement of the anal sphincter and anal mucosa.

Causes

−Assisted delivery.

−Prolonged secong stage of labor.

−Nulliparity.

−Macrosomia.

−Occipito-posterior position.

Complications

−PPH.

−Injury to bladder, uterus.

−Anal incontinence.

−Infections.

−Dyspareunia.

Management

−Surgical repair of the tear.

−Repair of the external anal sphincter end to end and internal inner sphincter should be repaired by interupted sutures.

−Repair of the 3rd and 4th perineal tear should be done in theatre under general or regional anesthesia.

−Its recommended to repair perineal tears with vicryl 2-0 which causes less irritation and discomfort.

−Check the anal canal if it is not closed during the repair.

−Antibiotics and laxatives are recommended to be used after anal sphincter repair.

−Women with history of anal sphincter injury in previous pregnancy who are symptomatic should be advised about elective CS.

POSTPARTUM HEMORRHAGE (PPH)

Definition

−Loss of more than 500 ml of blood from the genital tract in the first 24 hours after vaginal delivery and more than 1000 ml after CS.

−Excessive vaginal bleeding resulting in signs of hyovolemia (hypotension, tachycardia, oliguria, light headedness).

−A 10% decline in postpartum hemoglobin concentration from the antepartum levels.

Types

−Primary: within first 24 hours.

−Secondary: after 24 hours to the end of puerperium.

Risk Factors

−Overdistension of the uterus (polyhydramnios, multiple pregnancies, macrosomia…).

−Grand multiparity.

−Previous history of PPH.

−Antepartum hemorrhage.

−Myomatous uterus.

−Hypertensive disorders.

−Drug use (MgSo4, salbutamol…).

Causes

–Atonic uterus (70%).

–Genital tract trauma (20%).

–Retained placenta or placental fragment (10%).

–Coagulopathy (1%).

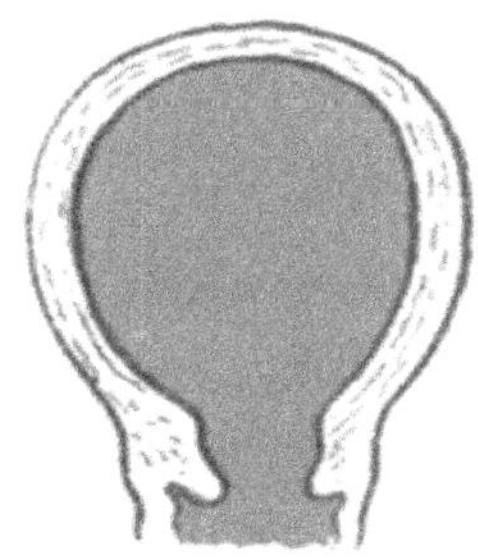

Atonic Uterus

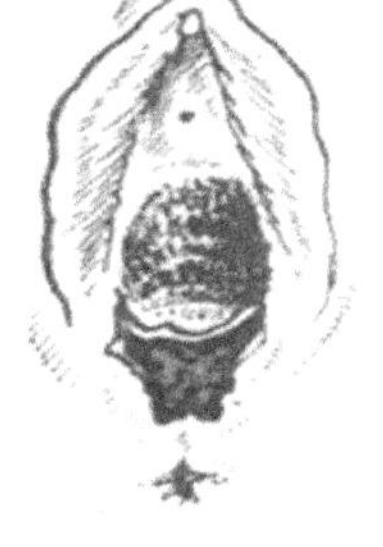

Genital Tract Trauma

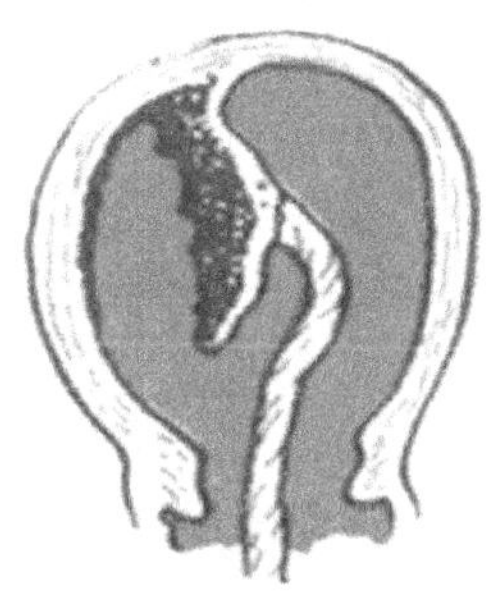

Retained Placenta

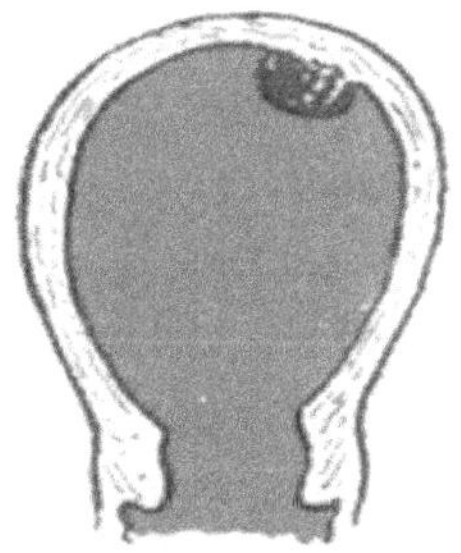

Retained Placental Fragment

Diagnosis

–Continuous vaginal bleeding.

–Signs of hypovolemic shock.

–Signs of anemia.

<u>Complications</u>

−Hypovolemic shock.

−Sheehan syndrome.

−Renal failure.

−Anemia.

−Death.

<u>Management</u>

−Call for help (obstetrician, anesthesist…).

−Resuscitation of the mother.

−Identification of the specific cause of PPH.

−Atonic uterus: bimanual compression and ecbolics (oxytocin, methyl ergometrin, misoprostol).

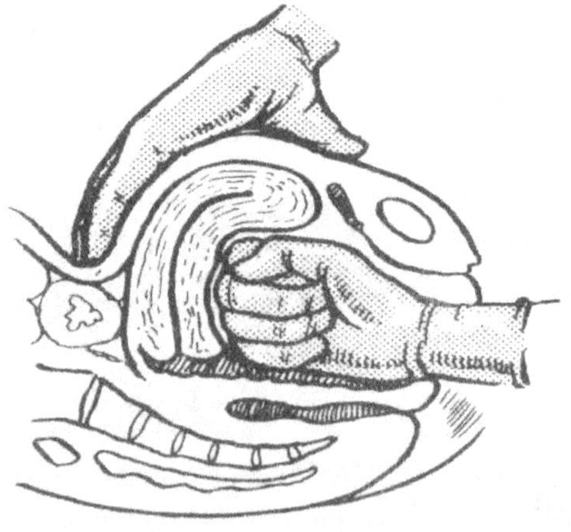

Bimanual Compression of the Uterus

−Genital tract trauma: vaginal exploration and repair under anaesthesia.

−Retained placenta or placental fragment: manual removal under anaesthesia.

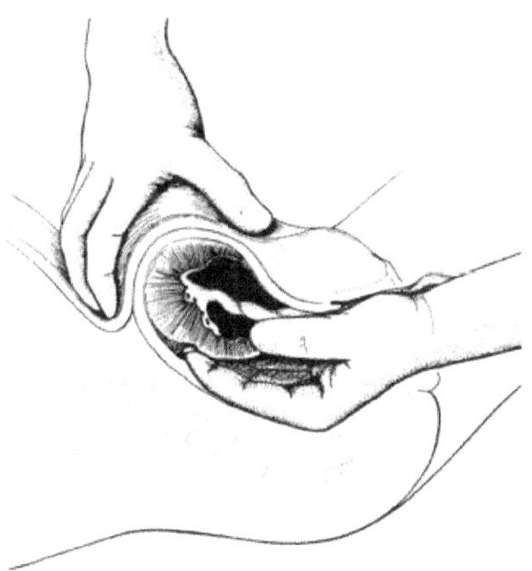

Manual Separation of the Placenta

−Coagulopathy: fresh frozen plasma, fresh blood transfusion, cryoprecipitate, fibrinogen, and platelet concentrate.

−If bleeding persists: internal iliac artery ligation or hysterectomy (standard procedure if bleeding is uncontrollable).

INSTRUMENTAL VAGINAL DELIVERY

Definition

Operative vaginal delivery is extraction of baby with use of instruments (obstetric forceps and vacuum extractor).

Indications

<u>Fetal</u>

−Fetal distress.

<u>Maternal</u>

−Prolonged second stage of labor.

−Maternal exhaustion.

Prerequisite for Instrumental Delivery

−Full dilatation of cervix.

−Engagement of fetal head.

−Empty the urinary bladder of the patient.

−Favorable presentation (vertex, deflexed vertex or face presentations).

−Vacuum extraction is contraindicated for face presentation.

−Vaccum extraction is contraindicated before 34 weeks of gestation.

−Instrumental delivery with high suspicion of failure should be done in theatre ready for CS.

−Episiotomy is not routenly indicated with instrumental delivery.

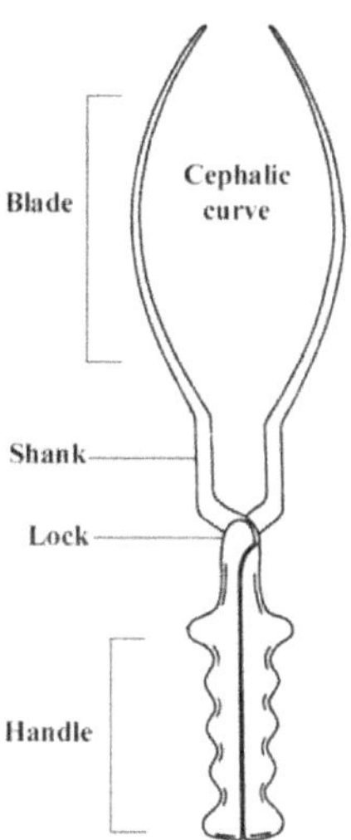

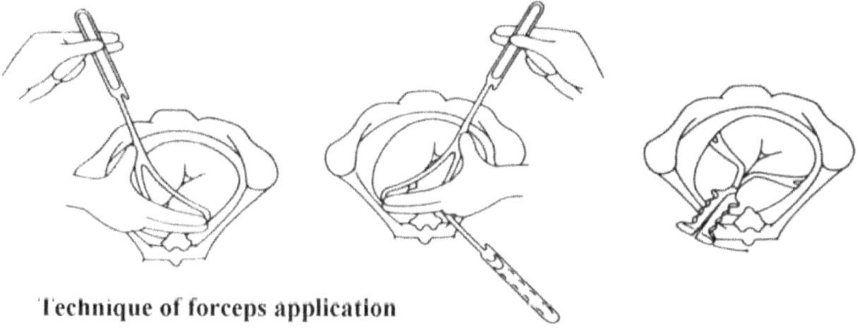

Technique of forceps application

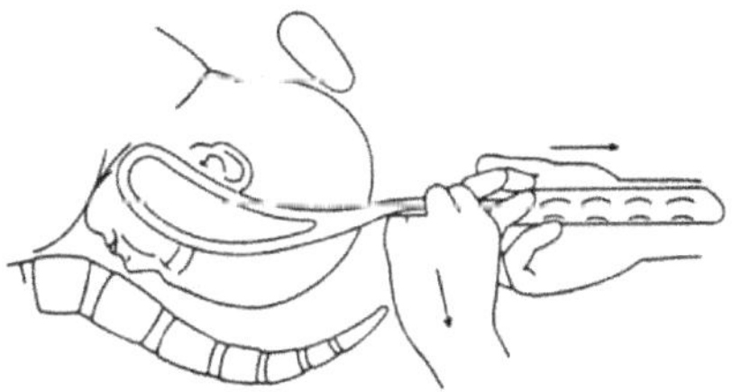

Direction of traction

Obstetric Forceps

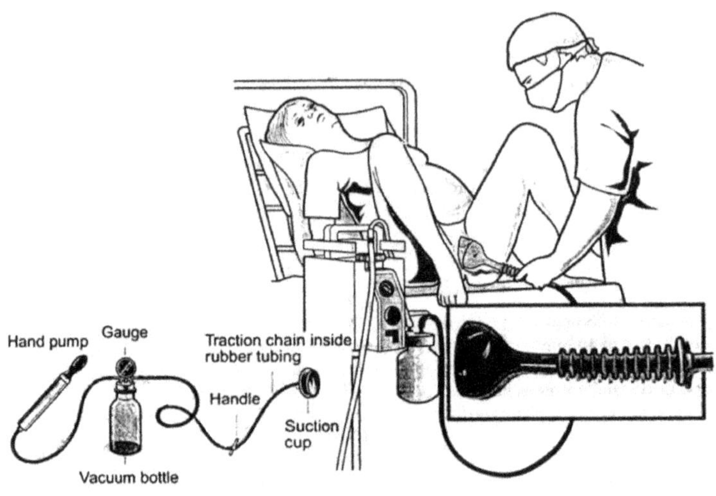

Vacuum Extractor

Complications

<u>Maternal</u>

−Traumatic injury including anal sphincter and bladder damage.

−Postpartum hemorrhage.

<u>Fetal</u>

−Skull fracture and/or intracranial hemorrhage.

−Cephalhematoma.

−Facial nerve injury.

−Facial skin bruises and lacerations.

<u>CESAREAN SECTION (CS)</u>

<u>Definition</u>

Delivery of the fetus, placenta and membranes through abdominal and uterine incisions after viability.

<u>Indications</u>

<u>Maternal</u>

−More than one previous CS.

−Contracted pelvis.

−Obstructive tumors.

−Abnormal uterine action.

−Medical conditions, eg, hypertensive disorders, diabetes mellitus, cardiac, pulmonary, thrombocytopenia.

−Reconstructive vaginal surgery, eg, fistula repair.

−Abdominal cerclage.

−Active genital herpes virus.

<u>Fetal</u>

−Fetal distress.

−Cord prolapse.

−Malpresentations.

−Macrosomia, congenital anomalies, multiple pregnancy.

<u>Maternal-Fetal</u>

−Maternal-fetal disproportion.

−Obstructed labor.

−Placenta praevia.

−Placental abruption.

−Perimortem.

Types

−Lower segment CS (more common).

−Upper segment CS.

Technique

<u>Pre-operative</u>

−Patient consent.

−Laboratory investigations.

−Anesthesia consultation: regional anesthesia is preferred than general anesthesia.

−NPO when elective CS.

−Intravenous: ringer lactate or normal saline 500 ml.

−Monitoring vital signs.

−Urinary bladder catheterization.

−Antibiotics.

Operative

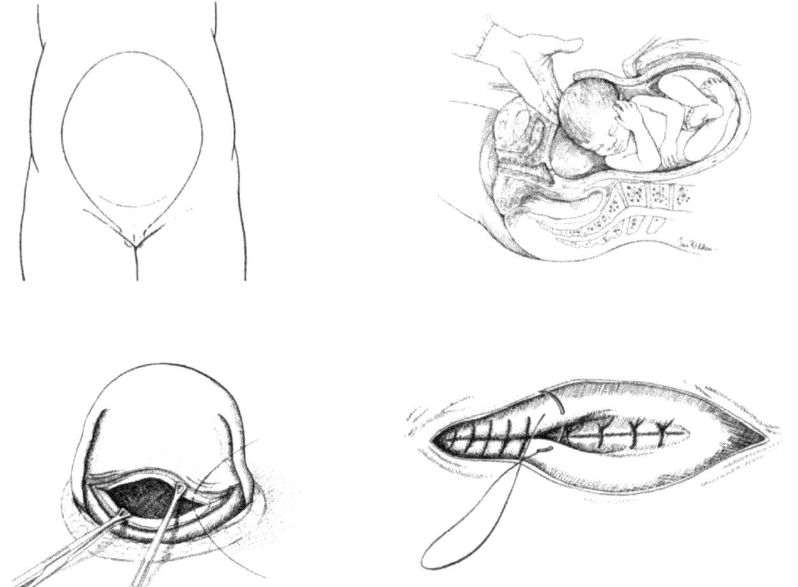

Post-operative

−Monitoring of vital signs and fundal status every 4-8 hours for 24 hours.

−Uterus massages and report extra lochia.

−Monitor fluids intake and output every four hours for 24 hours.

−Encourage early activity.

−Give fluids and soft diet after 6 hours.

−Antibiotics if indicated.

−Pain relief medication.

−If Rh incompatibility, administer anti-Rh immunoglobulin.

−Discuss infant feeding and contraception.

Complications

−Anesthesic complications.

−Hemorrhage and shock.

−Urinary tract injury.

−Gastrointestinal injury.

−Lacerations.

−Post operative peritonitis.

−Endometritis.

−DVT and PE.

−Paralytic ileus, acute gastric dilatation, and intestinal obstruction.

−Abdominal adhesions.

−Intrauterine synechia.

−Uterine dehiscence / rupture in the next pregnancy.